Anti-Inflammatory Diet

3 Step Guide for Beginners on How to Reduce Inflammation, Gain Energy, and Heal the Immune System

An Easy Cookbook, 2-Week Meal Plan & Top 50 Anti-Inflammatory Foods

Rebecca Barton

Tables of Contents

Introduction

Food provides our body with the nutrition it needs to carry out every life processes that are needed to survive. Food goes through a complete digestive system to be broken down and absorbed into the bloodstream so you can get all the energy all day long. Food also helps build our new cells and heal any wounds or affected wounds. Diet is a pattern of food calories and portions consumed by people of different ages based on their body needs and wants. There are countless diets you could find on the internet or in books; nowadays, many articles talk about that online too. A diet can be big or small, depending on what the specific need is. Different diets serve different purposes. Diets can be healthy for an individual and unhealthy for another one at the same time. In this growing world of junk food and ready meals, the overall disease rate has risen faster than usual, which can also be chronic or fatal.

The only way to be saved from all diseases is to adopt a healthy lifestyle that may look difficult at first, but when someone gets used to a healthy lifestyle, the benefits are so promising that one hardly ever returns. That, one cannot control; but food plays an important role in this. That does not mean that there is no way in which the risk cannot be minimized.

Everyone is generally aware of the different food groups, their benefits, and what is better and what is not. There is a part in which it should be consumed. Diet is not a limitation, but it is a way that can lead to a happier life and a better lifestyle. Many food chains have introduced much healthier options, and many people are turning their choices out of their interest to build a better lifestyle and body, with a growing awareness that people finally understand that a healthy body is a healthy mind.

A body only functions properly if sufficient nutrients are taken in. One should closely monitor and record their eating style and habit to know what they are consuming; with diet control and balance, one would never be obese and have the best of the body they could. Diet affects the body in different ways. It also affects the general reason why and what the body needs. As mentioned earlier, *not all diets are healthy*. Sometimes adopting a diet not necessary for the body can cause severe anxiety and eating disorders or some other problem in general.

We all grow up and listen about balanced diets. Not only this, we study it throughout our education system, and sometimes it is limited to just our education and not implemented in life, but that can also be quite disappointing. A balanced diet is one that consists of all the essential nutrients that help a person stay happy and healthy. When person absorbs the correct amount and servings, that is known as a balanced diet. The body must function properly. Eating a balanced diet helps with a healthy lifestyle, helps with a better life, and eliminates the risk of being sick. At the same time, physical health also affects mental health. Junk food is undoubtedly very tasty, which is why people are so overly fond of it and keep chewing it because it also feels good for our taste buds, and to satisfy the craving, we end up with a cheeseburger over a salad. Everyone has been there and enjoyed it too, but later the effects show that a salad was much better than a cheeseburger. The fat composition on the body generally starts to become visible if it is not taken into account early. Planning to eat a healthy diet isn't a problem, but sticking to a diet is. Humans always want to experience new things, especially in food, because of the taste buds who want something that is good for the tongue but bad for the body. Eating healthy helps in many ways. Sticking to a diet can be difficult, but some tips can help you ace what you want.

Step 1. Understand What Body Inflammation Is and How to Fight It

Don't Expect Too Much Too Soon

Always stay positive about the diet and don't expect sudden changes too soon. People are impulsive, and they want to change so quickly that they forget that a body has a full way of processing. One should not put pressure on oneself, and just go with the flow because that is what the body needs; under pressure, things start to cause fatigue. Give yourself and your body the time it needs. Don't jump to conclusions too early, and don't be discouraged when it takes time to reach someone's goal. Not everyone responds the same to the diet, and each individual has their own pace and speed.

Motivation

Motivation is the key to everything; there is nothing you can do if you are not motivated because if you lose motivation, it can be quite hectic. Motivation helps the person achieve more and do better, which is the most important thing. Always keep the purpose and importance in mind; otherwise, one would never do what is necessary for life. Losing hope and giving up is not an option, and diet is all about patience, which requires motivation, so one should always be motivated to do better and strive to do better. Motivation can be in any form. For example, after the end-of-week diet, you'll be surprised with a meal, perhaps a cheesecake that would serve the purpose and also motivate you because gifts and puffs help motivation.

Take Out the Junk

It can be very difficult to focus on healthy snacks and nutrition when there's junk food in the house; it is a distraction, and it can also happen when someone continues a healthy diet. You can't completely avoid it, but keep it out of sight. Once the clutter is out of sight, it can also be forgotten.

Eat a Jam Packed Breakfast

Eating a packed breakfast is very important. That's something that nourishes all day. If someone doesn't eat well in the morning, it can be quite hectic in the other 24 hours as well.

Know Your Body

A person should always understand the body and then decide what to eat. Not all food is the same for everyone, so always know what your body needs and then switch to a diet. This will help achieve better results and also stick to them.

What Is Body Inflammation?

Inflammation, in general, is a process by which cells in the body, such as white blood cells, protect the body from infection or other diseases that can attack, namely viruses or bacteria.

Inflammation can be reduced in several ways that help strengthen the immune system. It causes many chemical reactions and helps to find any kind of infection in the body. It also helps to increase blood flow in the body and also heals any broken muscles or tissues. It also generates the signal of pain, indicating that something is wrong in the body. Sometimes inflammation is also called fire—it is compared to it when the fire is often under control. In the form of heat or bonfire, it keeps us warm, healthy, and protected, but too much fire can be dangerous; it can also get out of control and cause many problems. It can also be destructive. It is not necessary for the fire to be present in a small amount to cause damage. It can also be a minor explosion that can affect. The mild inflammation helps to repair and maintain body tissues and muscles and also helps to generate healthy cells, but once their formation increases, it can cause many chronic diseases that can cause many problems.

Acute Infection

In fact, acute inflammation is shorter in duration and can last several minutes or days, depending on the injury.

Chronic Infection

Chronic inflammation occurs when the immune system does not respond properly, and the inflammatory chemicals are continuously released by the body.

Diseases Related To Inflammation

- Alzheimer's disease

- Asthma

- Cancer

- Bronchitis

- Chronic pain

- Type 2 diabetes

- Heart diseases

- Bowel diseases

When the body has too many inflammations, the usual way to find that out is by doing a C-reactive protein blood test.

What Is Anti-Inflammatory Diet?

For illness caused by inflammation such as rheumatoid arthritis, doctors say that no specifically assigned diet can reduce the chance of inflammation. Still, a diet consisting of fish, vegetables, olive oil, and other things will help reduce inflammation. The diet consisting of this base is also known as the Mediterranean diet. When a person suffers from a specific illness or problem, their eating habits not only change, but they can also notice many weight problems. Many medicines are already prescribed for inflammation, just as medicines are important, the diet also plays an important role. Doctors usually suggest an anti-inflammatory diet that can help reduce inflammation completely and reduce the chance of inflammation, or provide relief to people who suffer from it.

An anti-inflammatory diet is far from the healthiest diet, and even if it doesn't minimize the inflammation issue, it'll be the sub-strain of having it. Many people use medications to reduce inflammation, and common medications such as brutes and aspirin can help change the body's chemical reaction, but every drug has side effects. Our lifestyle choices and healthy diet options can reduce inflammation, and a lot of research is being done to test whether the anti-inflammatory diet helps, and it does. It has a profound change in the level of inflammation.

The anti-inflammatory diet requires many other changes in addition to the food changes, such as:

Other Changes You Should Make

Do Not Smoke

When someone smokes, cigarettes contain a lot of tobacco that is dangerous. There are no tobacco products that would be safe. It consists of acetone-nicotine and carbon monoxide, which, when inhaled, damages the lungs and can also affect the entire body. Smoking can cause many complications in the body in the long term.

It damages not only the lungs but also the heart. It also damages the central nervous system; tobacco ingredients have a mood-altering drug known as nicotine. When it reaches the brain then, it makes you feel a little hyped for a while, but after that, a person always remains tired, and craving for more cigarettes that can damage the lungs and cause many infections. In people who smoke a lot, it can be cause of more chronic inflammation in their body. It can also cause tuberculosis and lung cancer. It also damages the whole cardiovascular system because the blood vessel starts to tighten, and then it shrinks, and the blood does not flow through it properly; and because the blood does not flow through it, the blood pressure rises, which can also cause damage to blood vessels.

Smoking can affect cardiovascular health, but it also affects the people around the user because not only does the person inhale, but the people around them also inhale. They are bad for both similarly: a non-smoker can also start to show some skin changes, such as the structure of the skin through smoking and tobacco starts to change, the fingernails and foot nails are immune to shock, but they can also cause fungal nail infections. It can also cause hair loss in people who soak. It also increases the risk of oral cancer, and they have a higher chance of developing pancreatic cancer and type 2 diabetes with more complications.

Smoking can be very difficult, but with a good plan and proper motivation, a person can make the decision and then go for therapies and quit once and for all.

Limiting Alcohol

Alcohol affects slowly and gradually. However, the effect starts as soon as a person takes a step; drinking wine is good for health, but for an alcoholic, it can have a huge effect on the body. Drinking a lot of alcohol can trigger the activation of digestive enzymes, mainly produced in the pancreas.

These enzymes can lead to inflammation, which can lead to serious complications like inflammatory liver damage. The liver is an organ that helps eliminate harmful substances from the body. Long-term alcohol can accelerate the use of the damage, and this process can also increase the risk of chronic liver inflammation and also cause scar tissue that destroys the liver, and other diseases that are life-threatening and can lead to many toxins. Toxins in the body can be very harmful. However, compared to men, women's bodies are more likely to consume more alcohol and take longer to actually digest.

The pancreas in the body helps to secrete insulin, and then they respond to glucose when the pancreas and liver are not functioning properly, it can cause low blood sugar, and it can cause an excessive amount of sugar in the pancreas. It can also affect the nervous system, one of the easiest ways to tell when we consume alcohol is that we have speech delay. We don't know what you do and where we are. We are taken completely out of our senses, this indicates that alcohol can damage once the central nervous system.

Train

Regular exercise is very important, and one cannot ignore its benefits. Exercise helps control weight. Many people complain a lot about weight gain. Exercise aids weight loss when a person burns calories to enhance their physical appearance. A person that cannot go to the gym but always does the exercise in their home and it gives them the same benefits as those in the gym, it also helps to fight against health problems and diseases, be it a metabolic syndrome, high blood pressure or another type of diabetes, depression, anxiety it also improves the physical appearance, and the activity sends out various brain chemicals making a person feel happier and relaxed and rested as exercise reduces stress and gives the body the energy it needs.

It also stimulates physical exercise early in the morning because for people who need the energy. It also promotes better sleep; that is when there is a physical activity, and people sleep faster and deeper. With good exercises, a person can also have better productivity and can also stay fit because they are more active compared to a person who does not train.

Sleep Well

People get better productivity and concentration from a good night's sleep, and it can increase the productivity and concentration. It also reduces the risk of weight gain because when a person does not sleep well, their chances of gaining weight increase as it is necessary to sleep 6 to 8 hours to keep fit. It is also said that people who have not slept well can also have fatigue and stress and can remain anxious all day. People who sleep well have a better athletic performance because they have more energy, have better coordination, and a better mental functioning.

Maintain Weight

Maintaining weight is very important because the amount of weight gained in this way can cause many health complications. The factors strongly affect our health in our body, causing many diseases such as cardiovascular disease, diabetes, cancer, asthma, cataracts, and fertility. The weight within the healthy range is fine, but if the weight is greater than that, it can cause a lot of problems and no one wants that. Being overweight can also cause heart disease. A person can stay lazy all day but some people genetically have a lot weight, but it can also be controlled with the right medications. Being lazy causes physical inactivity.

An anti-inflammatory diet consists of all the nutrients that the diet can suggest. They are high in fruits and vegetables, beans, nuts, fish, herbs, and spices.

What Should One Eat And Avoid?

What we eat affects the inflammation in our body, the anti-inflammatory diet, as the name says, it helps reduce pain and other inflammation symptoms. It can reduce up to 60% of the inflammation in the body. Not only does this diet help reduce the chances of you getting it, but it can also prevent them from getting worse.

This diet includes a high intake of fat consumption, mainly from olive oil, intake of omega-three fatty acids. It is a traditional diet because it has no processed foods.

Fruit and Vegetables

One of the easiest ways to make the diet healthy and colorful is to add fruits and vegetables, and it is also said to be necessary for a healthy diet. They are magical when it comes to lifelong health benefits. Fruits and vegetables help lower the risk of heart disease and help control blood pressure in the body. It helps lower cholesterol in the body and also reduces heart disease. It is said to be a way of minimizing cardiovascular problems. Cancer is one of the deadliest diseases, and no one wants to go through that. Fruits and vegetables also help reduce the risk of obesity. Eye vision is a complete blessing; normal or extreme vision can be controlled by including fruits and vegetables in the diet. It helps with a better digestive system and also helps with diabetes.

All vegetables and colorful fruits help fight inflammation. Eating a colorful, balanced diet that is high in fruits and vegetables contains phytochemicals and antioxidants that are said to be powerful anti-inflammatory nutrients, especially green, orange, yellow, red, and purple vegetables, and fruits contain these pigments more. The more people consume it, the better it is. At least 4 ½ cups a day is the right amount. More emphasis should be placed on vegetables compared to fruit. Kale, broccoli, and cabbage are also said to be high in vitamin K.

Whole Grain

The consumption of whole grains helps to make the diet healthier and better. Whole grains are high in protein, fiber, and other antioxidants. It reduces the risk of inflammation.

A recent study states that it prevents inflammation and its effects. Even consuming whole grains in a small portion helps increase good bacteria in the body and aids system-wide inflammation. We often want to lose weight, which means we drop carbohydrates to lose pounds. It reduces the risk of cardiovascular disease by 40%, which is great in the age of junk and fatty food consumption. It has a rich source of B vitamins and magnesium that help a strong heart and muscles. It also controls diabetes. Foods made from whole grain are a great source of fiber, they have complex carbohydrates that are good for the body, they are great for weight management, and they help control cancer. It also promotes a good digestive system. They provide long-lasting energy and more nutrients compared to others. They also stabilize blood sugar levels. The antioxidants in it are best for inflammation.

Unlike simple carbohydrates, rice, white pasta, and flour, they have blood sugar spikes that can help reduce physical stress, and for the knowledge, these carbohydrates are slowly digested compared to others, but this is good for the body as it keeps the sugar level under control. The energy level is always intact, and the metabolism is fine. It has fibers that help slow digestion and helps regulate blood sugar, and it also lasts a long time. Eating a healthy diet is very important for a healthy lifestyle.

Fish

Long-chain foods of omega-three fatty acids are good for reducing inflammation. One should eat at least two servings of fatty fish, namely mackerel, trout, sardines, etc. They have omega acids, which are a great way. Fish is high in protein and has many health benefits; it is low in fat compared to any other animal protein.

Omega 3 fatty acids are said to be good fats. The human body cannot synthesize it on its own, so they have to eat fish during their meals. It helps maintain heart and cardiovascular health by helping to prevent blood clotting and also helps prevent vasoconstriction. It is also a very good prenatal and postnatal neurological development in humans. It helps reduce tissue inflammation and prevents irregular heartbeat. It also helps reduce fatigue and anxiety. Besides fish, another way can also be fish oil supplements, it prevents hunger, and it also has vitamin D and calcium. Vitamin D aids in mental development and also regulates the functioning of the immune system. Calcium in fish aids in bone development. Iron is beneficial for blood formation and is also very important for pregnant women. Iodine is generally found mainly in fish that help fight the thyroid gland.

It is nutritious. Fresh fish should be preferred over canned or frozen fish because they lack the coating and the same nutrition as fresh fish. Heart attacks and strokes are the most common form of death in humans today, and eating fish can reduce the risk of heart disease and strokes. It is also very crucial for eye development, and breastfeeding and pregnant women should consume it for the proper development of the baby. Mercury should be avoided, however. Mental decline in a stressful environment is natural, but to avoid this, one should eat fish because it also prevents Alzheimer's disease. It is also said to treat depression.

Moderate Dairy Intake

Sometimes whole milk and non-fermented dairy products can

cause inflammation that is not good for the body; however, the effect can be very minimal, yet it increases inflammation, so it is better to have it in a controlled way rather than cardiovascular disease. One should reduce butter, cream, whole dairy products in their diet. They should take yogurt in a moderate amount because it is said to be anti-inflammatory.

Meat Consumption Rule (Red)

People who consume a lot of red meat have a greater problem with diabetes and cardiovascular disease, and many cancer-related diseases. Processed meat or red meat, such as hot dogs, steaks, and sausages, can play the largest role in the diseases. However, it is a good source of protein and iron, but it is not the best to consume as it increases inflammation. It is a muscle made from a bovine lamp or another mammal that sits on it, and red meat is a good source of certain nutrients such as iron and vitamin B12, and the human body needs these nutrients to have good blood formation and to produce red blood cells. It is also very high in the growth of enzymes and building muscles, bones, and other tissues, but red meat can cause many health problems, the most common being heart disease, kidney problems and digestive problems.

A lot of research states that eating red meat can lead to many diseases. Many of the researchers also believe that people with many heart conditions suffer from them due to the consumption of red meat, mainly because a lot of saturated fat has more red meat saturated fat than any other protein, be it the first chicken or legumes, saturated fats from any source are bad for the human body because it encourages many diseases that may not be good for us, it increases the chances of chronic diseases, and once it happens it is very difficult to go back to where it all started, it is better that people reduce red meat consumption and focus more on another source of nutrients such as fish because they are relatively less harmful compared to red meat.

Processed Food

The process can often cause reverse drift, which means most of the food we eat is processed differently, but there is a difference between mechanical processing and chemical processing. Mechanical processing does not involve chemicals, such as chemical-processing chemicals.

They are not the pure form of the four. The processed foods are high in sugar. It is very good for health. Drinks can lead to a lot of harmful diseases. Sugars are known as empty calories because they don't contain any nutrients of calcium that the body needs, it is just an energy source when taken. It can also cause increased heart disease and cancer, and destroy human metabolism, it can lead to diabetes, one of the chronic diseases; most people who consume sugar can be obese and therefore they cannot do much life progress and then they are not active in their daily life. Processed food is bad in any form whether it be sausage or hot dogs, it is very good for our taste buds and we often consume in huge amount. People always want to eat food that is good, but they don't look at the medical effects of the food, our appetite is mainly attracted to the food which is very sweet, salty and greasy, as this food contains the most energy and nutrients, and we need this to survive, but it is completely why in today's world the competition of food is so high that people generally fight for resources.

It is very rare that people eat well. It also causes a lot of brain damage, and it can make a person depressed and also cause fatigue. When we locate processed foods, we see that they contain many official chemicals that are not good for the body because everything that is taken artificially and other than the medical processes is wrong for the body and health. It consists of preservatives, taste. Preservatives are completely chemically unacceptable for the body. Processed foods are high in carbohydrates. Carbohydrates are a good source of energy, but they cause many diseases, as well as processed foods which are high in carbohydrates and are found in many varieties—one of the problems with processed foods is that they don't have the right balance between the nutrients and vitamins and due to the high sugar level of the carbohydrate content, blood sugar levels can excrete and cause diabetes, they are very low in nutrients and they do not have the right nutrients that our body needs they only have fiber that is good for the direction of processed food, but it is not good for regular intake when eating processed food. Processed foods are easy to cook because of the easy digestion and less fat and they do not provide the human body with the necessary energy to survive so people should cut the processed food from their lives once a week or once a month; twice a month is okay.

They have a lot of healthy fats, it consists of an excessive amount of Omega 6 fatty acids that cause inflammation in the body and people who consume these types of oils have a very increased risk of heart disease, these fats are hydrogenated, and it is stated in the research that hydrogenated fats are the unhealthiest fats.

Super Sweet

Excess sugar can be quite bad for your health. Sugar has devastating health effects. Sugar can speed up glucose levels, and it can cause diabetes if there is a lot of sugar in the body that can cause mood swings. It can cause anxiety and also severe headaches, also called migraine. People who avoid sugar are said to have fewer mood swings and less hormonal imbalances.

They are more energetic compared to people who take in a lot of excess sugar because they are emotional and balanced, and they are always lazy to work. Excess sugar can increase the risk of diabetes, and it can also make a person fat, when a person starts eating sugar, they don't realize how much they have eaten because it feels good on the stomach and appetite, but excessive sugar can increase blood sugar and contribute to the risk of type 1 and type 2 or type 3 diabetes.

These effects can cause a lot of nutrition defects in a body, it can also eliminate the need for other nutrients because the body seems the full immune system is severely damaged by the sugar.

When a person is sick, the body will fight with the germs, but because of too much sugar, it is also said that the sugar can also prevent the body from fighting the germs as it is supposed to fight bacteria and they actually feed on sugar, so when there is an excess of glucose in the body, these organisms cause infections which means that instead of the body being immune to diseases, it can be susceptible to these diseases and no one likes a sick body. No one can stop sugar but they can control the amount they take, but can also lead to a shortage of chromium.

Many people don't know this, but a chromium deficiency is caused by refined sugar that we take in a tea, coffee, or in a regular dessert. No one wants to grow old early; no one likes agents, especially if it's too early because sugar in the body can cause premature aging. Everyone knows that sugar can affect body composition, but they can also affect how the skin looks. It can also cause many breakouts on the skin and cause acne, and it is one of the main causes of acne: excess sugar because the skin can lose its elasticity and cause premature aging.

Everyone loves their teeth because it is one of the physical manifestations of the body. Once the body gets sugar, everyone knows that digestion starts in the mouth, excessive sugar can cause tooth decay. It is the life-threatening effect of sugar one can have, the cosmetic damage sugar causes tooth decay faster than any other nutrient, it is very important to take care of their teeth and to remove sugar from your diet. A small amount of sugar is needed daily to satisfy the appetite, but adopting many ways and ways of exercise can be very bad. Many people are not aware that heart disease is often caused by gum disease, it can lead to inflammation in the body that lead to dental problems, and dental problems lead to a fast path to heart disease, many people believe that when body has an inflammatory response, it is also limited because of too much sugar, everyone has to adjust a healthy lifestyle to reduce the risk of chronic inflammation, so it is necessary to reduce the risk of a greater and more serious health condition.

Sugar also leads to stress when we are in stress mode and when a person is not mentally stable, and under pressure, under depression, our body goes into battle mode and starts releasing many hormones in the same way it happens when the sugar level in the blood is low, that's why people who consume more sugar seem to have been hyperactive which is medically not good as it can cause anxiety later on and also cause body shocks. It can also cause high levels of fructose in the body that can damage the liver, and when fructose is broken down it converts to fat, it can also damage our pancreas, and the pancreas may not make insulin because they are sure that if a person eats a lot of sugar, they will control its role; otherwise the pancreas starts to make more insulin, and this will go over the pancreas, and it can get type 2 diabetes.

Use of Olive Oil

Today there are a lot of oil on the market that is used for cooking such a sunflower oil. The best oil is the extra virgin olive oil. When it comes to cooking research, it shows that the extra virgin olive oil is not only the excellent choice, but it is also great for cooking as it has to lower blood pressure and regulate cholesterol levels, which are the main problem of inflammation in the body.

Olive oil can be used for any purpose, whether it's salad dressing or for general use. Anything that contains olive oil contains monounsaturated fatty acids, and it occurs in many grapes, whether it will be called pure virgin or extra virgin oil. It is not as processed as other oils and has a lot of phytochemicals that are good for cooking. It is naturally extracted from olive oil; it contains only 14% saturated fat, it is 11% polyunsaturated fatty acid that is omega-3 fatty acids.

Olive oil has strong anti-inflammatory properties, which is a great source in the anti-inflammatory diet and helps treat many of the diseases mentioned above. Extra virgin olive oil can help to minimize the effect of inflammation and therefore, it is one of the healthiest oil. One of the ways in which the effects of inflammation are minimized is by antioxidants that the oleic acid has, which is the large supply of antioxidants caused when there is an obstruction in blood flow in the heart or brain and is the cause of a blood clot, and then strokes occur as one of the second most common causes of death after a heart attack.

Olive oil helps minimize strokes. People who consume olive oil are less prone to strokes and heart disease than the people who use sunflower oil. The risk of suffering from heart disease was lower in the Mediterranean countries. The level of inflammation is low, and it helps minimize altitude sickness, which helps to lower blood pressure, and it also stops pain and death.

Olive oil in the food prevents the person from becoming

depressed and helps to stay active for the improvement of life processes and, if not cared for, it can cause depression, but olive oil is said to help fight depression. It also helps with any problems with metabolic deficits that occurred in the body. In the current era, breast cancer is the most common cancer in every woman. Extra virgin oil will fight breast cancer.

Minimizing the risk of breast cancer is very good for women and children, and brain development is essential for children. Olive oil has the most powerful antioxidant known as polyphenol, which helps reverse the oxidative damage that helps a person with aging.

Likewise, olive oil also helps prevent skin cancer when there is also a lot of dangerous cancer, with deficient nutrients regularly causing cancer and various parts of the body. Skin cancer is one of the most dangerous cancers, so olive oil is over and helps oxidize the effect of the sun, and similarly, it prevents skin cancer. Especially in women, there is a lot of joint pain and bone fractures, so that diet that helps. Olive oil supplements also found in pharmacies aid in the treatments of bones, osteoporosis, which occurs especially in postmenopausal women. So if olive oil is consumed throughout life, it can also minimize the likelihood of its diminution and also help keep the person alive and young, as it is not known that dietary olive oil helps the heart to stay healthy and function properly. The heart is also going through an aging process, and over time the blood vessels and blood vessels may not work the way they do for a child. Using stored olive oil prevents aging physically and internally.

Use of Coconut Oil

When cancer has frequently occurred, a different inflammatory disease is so common that many people use the coconut oil. Coconut oil increases HDL cholesterol, and LDL cholesterol decreases, which helps keep cholesterol in the body under control.

People who consume coconut oil are often told that it does not cause damage; it is important to take coconut oil in the diet as extra virgin coconut oil has anti-inflammatory properties that help fight inflammation.

Who Should Take an Anti-Inflammatory Diet?

Anti-inflammatory food reduces inflammation in the body, and it is a type of diet also known as one-size-fits-all because it can be followed by people of any age with symptoms because it is such a great and complete package diet that does not eliminate key nutrients, but also accelerates the effects of each nutrient in a single diet and removes excess harmful nutrients given or present from the body.

The correct amount of diet needed is most closely related to the Mediterranean diet—a diet adopted by some other Mediterranean countries, it is like a traditional diet and does not need to be followed by a certain age group. It does not only prevent the person from getting inflammatory diseases but also minimizes the chance that it happens in your body; if a child follows an anti-inflammatory diet from a very young age, they will not suffer from inflammatory diseases in the future.

Just the pattern of a balanced diet with the right amount of nutrients and the right amount of food portions is said to make you less prone to chronic inflammatory diseases, it is not a diet to lose weight, it is not a diet to lose anything, but a diet to lead a healthy lifestyle, it can be adapted for a better lifestyle to be better and to work better, but you should always consult a nutritionist before starting a diet.

What Are the Effects on the Body if the Person Does Not Take an Anti-Inflammatory Diet?

People who do not follow anti-inflammatory diets are more susceptible to diseases that can be caused to them. Inflammation is bad in the body, causing the immune system to malfunction and cause many chronic diseases known as chronic inflammation, and the body will not fight against other diseases and will be more attractive to various germs and bacteria, the cells will not generate properly.

There will be joint pain, and the person may have strokes, or they may also become depressed because inflammatory affects both mental health and physical health. The anti-inflammatory diet is not a regimen, but it is a way of adjusting a certain lifestyle, a certain way of eating. The Mediterranean diet is one of the examples of an anti-inflammatory diet. It is not something that would harm the body. In fact, the body benefits from its nutrients, and it also helps the body because what we eat every day has different effects on the body and everything reacts differently.

The anti-inflammatory diet contains food that increases the benefits and reduces inflammation in the body, when people are not following an anti-inflammatory diet and continue to chew sugar and processed food, it can worsen inflammation that can last the person a lifetime. An anti-inflammatory diet consists of many antioxidants, phytochemicals that help the body grow and fight against foreign germs. It helps to remove free radicals from the body and help the metabolism to work well. The people who could not follow anti-inflammatory diet have metabolic problems, the food is not digested properly, and symptoms are shown early because no one wants to get sick.

Everyone wants to lead a healthy lifestyle. Inflammation starts slowly but quickly grows in the form of diabetes, heart disease, stroke, cancer. All these deadliest diseases are caused if we don't adapt to a healthy lifestyle.

The anti-inflammatory diet follows a balanced diet that is essential for any human when there is inflammation in the body that would increase the risk of cell damage that a person did not take from the beginning, they should switch to medications, which helps to relieve the pain. The person suffering from a disease may be relieved by these drugs in the end, but it has other side effects that can damage the body in various ways. It is often said that medication is very easy to take, it does not require much effort, but the anti-inflammatory diet is a very easy to cook and easy to eat diet because it can be easily consumed by children of all ages.

People who are not on an anti-inflammatory diet may suffer from anti-inflammatory conditions bowel disease allocation metabolic syndrome that would cause type 2 diabetes, high blood pressure, cardiovascular disease and obesity inflammation play a role in all of these diseases, and an anti-inflammatory diet helps a person's health to improve. The anti-inflammatory diet is not expensive to follow.

Benefits of Anti-Inflammatory Diet

There are many benefits of following the anti-inflammatory diet, because an anti-inflammatory diet consists of many nutrients that benefit the body's boreal pathways in many ways.

Helps in Better Sleep

Sleep is very important to a person because when a person does not sleep well, they are simply irritated all day, and they may not be able to concentrate properly at work because they do not get 6 to 8 hours of sleep and cannot concentrate on everything because the brain is always tired, leaving a person unable to focus on anything. But this diet contains all the good nutrients that not only give the body what it needs but also give them a lot of energy. They work throughout day and night, we are so tired and stunned all day long that we always sleep well for 6 to 8 hours.

Sleeping 6 to 8 hours is very necessary for people of all ages to function properly because a body grows during sleep, and sleep is very important for the body's metabolic activities. It helps the person to get sound sleep.

People cannot have much caffeine or sugar, both sugar and caffeine wake people up and if there is a healthy lifestyle, adjusted in the right way with enough amount of nutrients in their life, sleep pattern is not disturbed whether it is a 1 hour 15-minute nap or a 6 to 8-hour sleep. Anti-inflammatory food helps in the peace of mind that promotes a good night's sleep.

Helps With Good Skin

The health of the skin is very important because it is a cosmetic appearance of the body, and it helps build confidence.

It also plays a very important role in many important tasks of the body. The skin protects the body against various viruses and bacteria, our skin is exposed to pollution and the outside world every. The anti-inflammatory diet is important because humans are exposed to sun and other UV rays which can be harmful to our bodies. We can get vitamin D from the sun, which helps to perform many other processes in the body by various organs, healthy skin also helps to maintain the temperature in the body because if the temperature is not maintained, this can cause many problems. Healthy skin helps to feel better.

The most common benefit of an anti-inflammatory diet is that it helps the skin—taking olive oil, coconut oil, fish oil which good fiber with low sugar content which is especially necessary for healthy skin. If there is a good diet, it is shown on the skin as it is the center of the body which consists of many fruits and vegetables that promote healthy skin and also cut away the sugar that makes the skin prone to acne and loosens elasticity because excess sugar can cause premature aging, wrinkles, and the skin loses its elasticity making it look very bad. Sometimes it can also cause skin cancer, so one has to adjust the anti-inflammatory diet because it not only grows the skin but it can also cause skin cancer.

Promotes Healthy Food

The inflammatory diet consists of vitamins, minerals, and other nutrients, and the overall diet strikes a good balance between carbohydrates, protein, sugar, and everything it contains. It also contains all the colorful fruits and vegetables needed for the body, so it promotes healthy eating and once adopted by people of all ages they need to eat healthy whatever it is it has a direct impact on the way they act, so the anti-inflammatory diet promotes healthy eating.

Reduces Inflammation

Inflammation can cause many diseases, and it also increases the risk of many chronic diseases. The benefit of an anti-inflammatory diet is that it reduces inflammation, which is the concept of any food crop and enough nutrients entering the body that releases antioxidants that help reduce information. It also prevents any further risk that may be caused by recovery and prevents any further risk that may be caused by inflammation.

Wide Range of Recipes

The anti-inflammatory diet is the most common type of diet. This diet is so popular and famous, it consists of thousands and thousands of recipes of all varieties. There is so much abundance of recipes that it is not necessary that people start from scratch, anyone can make them, no matter the number of people who live in a house, because the number of ingredients that are so readily available. It is a healthy diet. It's so easy and so convenient that they can start whenever and wherever they want, it's a very easy diet and can be followed by people of all ages. People on the internet do not hesitate before starting a diet because a healthy diet consists of a wide variety of foods, and that is what anti-inflammatory foods are all about.

Maintaining a Young Heart

An anti-inflammatory diet consisting of lots of fruits and vegetables and fewer fats and more monounsaturated fats and does not contain any of the foods that would lead to LDL cholesterol which will lead to a lot of composition of fat on people which also affects the heart.

Fight Against Premature Aging

At the beginning of the method, it consists of nutrients and many other vitamins and minerals and also consists of polyphenols and antioxidants that prevent the body from premature aging because it maintains the elasticity of the skin, it also helps with various reasons that would cause aging in a certain person, an informative diet therefore also prevents premature aging.

Prevents Cancer

Cancer is one of the deadliest diseases in today's era, and many foods accelerate it. The anti-inflammatory diet is made up of many foods rich in vitamins, minerals, and nutrients that prevent cancer in people of all ages, not just one specific type of cancer or limited type, but different types of cancer, skin cancer, breast cancer, bone cancer, and blood cancer. It is completely based on a good and healthy lifestyle, and a healthy lifestyle does not produce cells that would multiply and cause cancer in such a way, it is a very good diet that promotes not only a healthy eating habit but also prevents various diseases such as cancer.

Prevents Joint Pain

Inflammation is one of the most common things that cause the joint pain that occurs with aging, so an inflammatory diet protects the joint and helps to keep fit and build stronger bones and muscles that don't cause bone disease like osteoporosis.

It provides the right amount of vitamins and nutrients needed for bone formation and health.

Helps Mental Health

The anti-inflammatory diet helps fight depression and will help you have good mental health in general, as it is said that a healthy body is a healthy mind. It mentally prepares the body to fight against any illness or any conditions. It consists of antioxidants that are set to fight depression. When a person is confident, the person is confident about everything, and self-confidence is always needed in a person. Oxidation mainly occurs, causing Alzheimer's disease.

Better Vision

One of the greatest blessings for humans is the anti-inflammatory diet that consists of many grains and legumes that contain vitamin A and helps with better vision; it also prevents the vision from becoming too weak, and from having blurred vision because it contains all fruits and vegetables.

Helps Indigestion

The anti-inflammatory diet is high in fiber, as we all know fiber aids in digestion, so the anti-inflammatory diet aids in better digestion and also maintains the body's metabolic rate for better digestion, the person digests food more easily, and it does not cause problems in the digestive tract, the food is always easily consumed and digested.

Maintains Blood Sugar Levels

The anti-inflammatory diet maintains blood sugar levels. The sugar that can be consumed is much less in this scenario. The blood sugar is always maintained so that it does not cause any kind of diabetes that can be caused by excess sugar and exceeding processed food.

Advantages and Disadvantages of Anti-Inflammatory Diet From the Medical Perspective

Not every diet is perfect, and not every diet gives the best results. Every diet has its advantages and disadvantages; likewise, the anti-inflammatory diet also has its advantages and disadvantages.

Advantages

Reduces Inflammation

When a person eats food that reduces inflammation and aids the immune system, it stops attacking every part of the body, and then it also begins to decline over time, and the body begins to recover. It is the only benefit from a medical point of view that the anti-inflammatory diet has started to reduce inflammation in the body.

Reduces Pain

It reduces pain caused by inflammation in the body.

Promotes Weight Loss

The biggest advantage of an anti-inflammatory diet is the weight loss that many people on a diet have to get the desired weight. The anti-inflammatory diet is not tasty, but it also helps with the weight loss system. It consists of everything constructive and is not limited to a different group, it only eliminates the harmful foods that are also beneficial to our health, it promotes weight loss in such a way that a person would lose weight without feeling low daily, but the diet is filled with energy, and a person does not feel fatigued or stressed when following it, it also allows sugar in the form of fruits and other dairy products, but in limited amounts, so it is the bigger and better way to reduce weight.

Cons

Consists of Many Allergens

The anti-inflammatory diet consists of many foods that can be allergenic to humans. Fish, almonds like nuts, not all people like this kind of diet. It consists of nuts that people usually do not tolerate, and that lead to allergies in the body, so it can be a bit of a pain for them.

Step 2. Avoid What Is Not Good for Your Body and Creates Inflammation

Foods to Eat and to Avoid

In fact, an anti-inflammatory diet is an eating plan designed to prevent and treat chronic inflammation, which further leads to many health problems. Chronic inflammation is the primary home for some of the major diseases and various health problems. In a typical anti-inflammatory diet, the focus is on lean proteins, fruits, nuts, vegetables, healthy fats, and seeds.

Factors That Cause Chronic Inflammation

Chronic inflammation is caused when the immune system releases the chemicals intended to fight the injuries, viruses, and bacterial infections, even in the condition where there are no intruders to fight with. This is mainly due to lifestyle factors, for example, taking the stress and lack of exercise.

Health Benefits of an Anti-Inflammatory Diet

The fact is that the food we choose to eat directly affects the level of inflammation in our body. An anti-inflammatory diet has the benefit of helping to treat chronic inflammation and also helping to prevent and treat the following diseases:

- Alzheimer's disease

- Asthma

- Arthritis

- Allergies

- Depression

- Cancer

- Gout

- Diabetes

- Heart disease

- Inflammatory bowel diseases, including Crohn's disease and ulcerative colitis

- Irritable bowel syndrome (IBS)

- Stroke

The Food You Should Eat During an Anti-Inflammatory Diet

The studies show that with a high intake of fruit, vegetables, nuts, seeds, fish, and healthy oils, you have a lower risk of diseases related to chronic inflammation. Also, substances such as the antioxidants and omega-3 fatty acids in some foods seem to have anti-inflammatory effects.

List of Foods High in Antioxidants

- Cherries

- Apples

- Berries, including raspberries, blueberries, and blackberries.

- Artichokes

- Avocados

- Sweet potatoes

- Vegetables should be dark green leafy vegetables, including kale, spinach, and kale

- Broccoli

- Beans, including red beans, black beans, and pinto beans

- Nuts, including walnuts, almonds, pecans, and hazelnuts

- Dark chocolate must contain at least 70 percent cocoa

- Whole grains, including oats and brown rice

List of Foods With Increased Content of Omega-3 Fatty Acids

- Walnuts

- Flaxseed

- Oily fish, including salmon, herring, mackerel, sardines, and anchovies

- Omega-3 enriched foods like milk and eggs

Researchers also suggest that certain culinary spices and herbs also help reduce chronic inflammation. These are:

- Ginger

- Garlic

- Turmeric

Foods to Avoid in an Anti-Inflammatory Diet

While the foods high in omega-3 fatty acids are quite useful for treating chronic inflammation, the foods high in omega-6 fatty acids are known to have increased production of inflammatory chemicals in the body.

The omega-6 fatty acid is a type of essential fatty acid that is present in various foods. Due to the fact that omega-6 fatty acids help regulate metabolism, keep bones healthy, and promote brain function, it is recommended not to completely cut the supply of omega-6 from your diet. You must balance the intake of omega-6 fatty acids with the intake of omega-3 fatty acids to control the level of chronic inflammation. The list of foods rich in omega-6 fatty acids is listed below.

- Meat

- Dairy products such as ice milk, butter, and cheese

- Margarine spread

- Vegetable oils should contain corn oil, safflower oil

- Soybean oil, peanut oil, and cottonseed oil

It is recommended to use oils such as avocado oil and olive oil instead of vegetable oils.

Aside from omega-6 intake and the preferred use of oil, it has also been suggested that people should avoid the use of sugary drinks, desserts, refined carbohydrates, and possessed snacks.

It is because the high intake of foods with a high glycemic index, such as refined grains and sugar, which are found in most owned foods and white bread, can accelerate inflammation levels.

Some Tips for Following and Maintaining an Anti-Inflammatory Diet

- Eat about five to nine servings of antioxidant-rich fruits and vegetables every day.

- Manage your intake of omega-6 fatty acids. Limit consumption of omega-6 fatty acids and increase the consumption of omega-3 fatty acids, including walnuts, flaxseed, and fatty fish such as tuna, salmon, herring, and mackerel.

- Manage your protein intake. Replace the protein sources for red meat with fish, lean poultry, soybeans, and lentils.

- Use olive oil, nuts, and seed oils in place of the vegetable oils and margarine because the former has the healthier benefits.

- Try to improve your taste by using anti-inflammatory herbs like ginger, garlic, and turmeric instead of flavoring your food with salt.

- Use the fiber-rich whole grains in place of refined grains like brown rice, quinoa, oats, pasta, which have the whole grain as the first ingredient and the bread.

Exercises You Should Take Before Starting an Anti-Inflammatory Diet

In addition to reversing a healthy diet, taking warm baths, and giving the nourishing massages, there is another way to reduce chronic inflammation, namely exercise. Before starting the anti-inflammatory diet, you should start exercising. Just 20 minutes of exercise a day can reduce your inflammation by 12%. The following types of exercise are best for reducing chronic inflammation.

Light Walk

Taking a light walk on a daily basis is the easiest and best way to reduce chronic inflammation. Walking helps your muscles recover, reduces inflammation by regulating fresh blood and oxygen throughout the body. It pumps the lymphatic system for the waste of removal.

Easy Walk

Aside from a light walk, easy walking is another way to restore your body and reduce inflammation. Immerse yourself in nature, find an easy path, join a friend or call one and go for easy hiking.

Foam Rolling Exercise

Exercise with foam rollers helps with muscle soreness, helps improve sleep and flexibility, aids digestion, and reduces chronic inflammation.

Yoga, Meditation, and Deep Breathing Exercise

If you want to reduce inflammation in the body, these tactics are the most common. These exercises help relax the mind and body, which is necessary to reduce inflammation.

These are the exercises that a person can perform before starting an anti-inflammatory diet and can also go through the diet. Since these are the lightest and most effective, everyone should include these exercises in their daily routine.

Step 3. Perform an Anti-Inflammatory Diet to Heal Your Body and Gain Energy

Healing your body inflammation and gaining more energy is never impossible. But an anti-Inflammatory diet is the way out to improve your immunity, fight against diseases, and make you gain more energy.

How Do You Find Easily Accessible and Affordable Anti-Inflammatory Ingredients?

All anti-inflammatory dishes are made with affordable nutritional components. If a person needs to follow an anti-inflammatory diet plan and can't keep up with the high-end nutritional component, a simple solution can be to stick to a clean and green diet, avoiding all kinds of continued foods and sugars. A nutritionist often advises that precautions are always better than regrets afterward. People who suffer from inflammatory diseases or diseases that can be caused by inflammation should follow a simple diet. The diet mentioned in the document is an easy diet and consists of components that are readily available and affordable for all classes. By critically analyzing the 14-day meal plan, it can be noted that morning and evening snacks consist of fruit that can be easily affordable in said amounts. In the future, it can be seen that the main dishes such as lunch and dinner also consist of vegetables in the form of salad. Protein is present on alternative days, as it is also considered a necessity for the proper functioning of a person's metabolism. Other than that, the included bread can be to your taste (white or brown) or if the individual is gluten tolerant or intolerant.

In summary, all components are easily accessible and included in the daily diet of an inflammatory patient. Not only patients but also healthy people should include similar food content in their daily meals to stay healthy and away from other diseases too.

A Quick Step by Step Procedure of an Anti-Inflammatory Diet

Aggravation allows the body to fight ailments and can protect it from pain. As a rule, it is an essential part of the re-cooperation procedure.

Nevertheless, a few people have a condition where the invulnerable frame does not fill properly. This interference can cause diligent or intermittent mild irritation. Persistent irritation occurs with various conditions, for example, psoriasis, rheumatoid joint inflammation, and asthma. There is evidence that dietary decisions can help with side effects.

A calming diet prefers products from the soil, nutrition with omega-3 unsaturated fats, whole grains, lean proteins, powerful fats, and flavors. It demoralizes or limits the use of prepared food and red meat.

The soothing diet is anything but a certain routine, but rather a way of eating. The Mediterranean eating regimen and the DASH diet are examples of a diet with fewer carbohydrates.

More and more about irritation here.

What Is a Soothing Diet?

The soothing diet contains thick plant food supplements and avoids treated food sources and meat. Some foods contain fixations that can cause or intensify aggravation. Sugary or treated foods can do this while they are crunchy, whole foods are more averse to having this impact.

A soothing diet focuses on new foods grown from the ground. Many plant foods are an acceptable source of anti-cancer drugs. A few dietary supplements, as it can cause the development of free radicals. Models contain foods that individuals bake in heated cooking oil more than once.

Dietary cell reinforcements are atoms in food that help expel free radicals from the body. Free radicals are the characteristic results of some real procedures, including digestion. Be that as it may, external elements, such as stress and smoking, can increase the number of free radicals in the body.

Free radicals can cause cell damage. This damage increases the risk of aggravation and can contribute to a range of diseases. The body makes a few cancer prevention agents that help remove these harmful substances, but strengthening the dietary cells also helps. A calming diet promotes foods rich in anti-cancer agents over and above those that increase free radical formation. Omega-Three unsaturated fats, which are available in smooth fish, can help reduce the number of flammable proteins in the body. Fiber can also have this impact, according to the Arthritis Foundation.

Types of Calming Food

Numerous famous weight control plans are now adhering to soothing standards.

For example, both the Mediterranean eating regimen and the DASH diet contains new products from the soil, fish, whole grains, and fats that are beneficial to the heart.

Irritation appears to be doing a job in cardiovascular disease but inquires about the suggestion that the Mediterranean eating regimen, with an emphasis on plant foods and powerful oils, may lessen the effects of aggravation on the cardiovascular framework.

Try our dinner plan for the Mediterranean eating regime here.

Who Could Help It?

A soothing diet can be a reciprocal treatment for some conditions that become more deplorable from incessant exacerbation.

The associated conditions include:

- Rheumatoid joint inflammation

- Psoriasis

- Asthma

- Eosinophilic esophagitis

- Crohn's condition

- Colitis

- Fiery bowel disease

- Lupus

- Hashimoto's condition

- Metabolic disorder

Metabolic disorder refers to a range of conditions that generally co-exist, including Type 2 Diabetes, weight, hypertension, and cardiovascular disease.

Researchers recognize that irritation plays a role in this. A soothing diet can, therefore, help improve the well-being of a person with a metabolic disorder. The most effective method is using food to enable your body to fight aggravation. The type of food you eat will affect your overall health, right? Find out how your diet affects irritation in your body and what it means for your well-being.

The term "soothing food" is widely used in subsistence discussions today. Anyway, for what reason is aggravation terrible to us anyway? Besides, what does diet have to do with it?

Irritation is part of your body's normal response to contamination or damage. It is the point at which your damaged tissue releases synthetic brews that advise white platelets to start fixing. Whatever the case, in some cases, irritation is of poor quality, spread all over the body and continuously.

This incessant irritation can harm your body. It can take on a task in the development of plaque in your pipes that can increase your risk of coronary disease and stroke. It is also linked to an increased risk of malignant growth, diabetes, and other incessant conditions.

Learn How Your Diet Is Helpful and How It Is Harmful

The decisions you make can affect the irritation in your body. Researchers have not yet figured out how diet affects the body's flammable procedures, but they know a number of things.

Research shows that what you eat can affect the amount of C-responsive protein (CRP) –a marker of worsening– in your blood. That could be because a few foods like prepared sugars help offload and can increase the danger of endless irritation. Various foods like leafy greens help your body fight against oxidative pressure, which can cause irritation.

The uplifting news: calming foods will generally be similar foods that can keep you healthy in different ways. So eating given irritation doesn't have to be complicated or priceless.

Clear, General Guidelines for Reducing Food

- **Eat more plants:** Whole plant supplements have the calming supplements your body needs. So eating a rainbow of organic products, vegetables, whole grains, and vegetables is the best place to start.

- **Focus on anti-cancer substances**: They help prevent, delay, or fix a number of types of cell and tissue damage. They are found in beautiful soil products such as berries, green vegetables, beets, and avocados, as well as beans and lentils, whole grains, ginger, turmeric, and green tea.

- **Buy your Omega-3s**: Omega-3 unsaturated fats have a job in controlling your body's inflammation procedure and can help manage pain identified with irritation. Locate these healthy fats in fish such as salmon, fish, and mackerel, as well as small amounts in pecans, walnuts, ground flaxseed, and soy.

- **Eat less red meat:** Focus on a reasonable goal. Try taking your afternoon burger a few times a week with fish, nuts, or soy-based proteins.

- **Cut the prepared things:** sugary oats and drinks, Southern-style foods, and baked goods are generally starred, provocative culprits. They can contain a lot of unfortunate fats related to aggravation. Either way, eating whole organic produce, vegetables, grains, and beans can be fast if you get the chance to eat countless meals.

Example of a girl who used the inflammatory process in her

difficult times.

I previously had skin inflammation in the seventh grade. For me, it meant that at the age of 12, the skin around my eyes became red, puffy, dry, and wiry–and as such, stayed on and off for a long time.

My primary care doctor and the dermatologists I later saw recommended a topical steroid cream. That stuff is generally not meant for long-term use, so I would try applying a little. At least it didn't take much. I just got used to applying a huge amount of cosmetics to distract individuals based on what happened to me.

At the time, a few years earlier, I went through the book The Plan by Lyn-Genet Recitas. It's an eating routine book that swears to work by reducing constant, poor quality food. Overall, I love health – I like to exercise and watch out for what I eat – so I chose to try it.

Her book says that specific "solid" foods are not likely to work for everyone. Previously, I worked with a fitness coach who urged me to eat meat and protein, just a huge amount of protein. Her book encourages that things like Greek yogurt or protein powder aren't really solid when it gives a chance that it makes your own extraordinary body feel awful. It's also real: when I tuned into my coach and focused on meat, my skin went wild.

I followed the book's three-week supper plan, and within a month, I dropped 15 to 20 pounds. I noticed that at every point I strayed from the precise diet she recommended, it would creep back up. The idea is to throw out all the provocative food, start with taking out meat and dairy products, and then gradually to take it back up. It was not difficult to eat so carefully; I thought I would be hungry all the time, but I wasn't. What was difficult was the time it took to be prepared for everything. That's where I got off the track. I just didn't have the chance.

At that point, a year ago, I chose to reread The Plan and accomplish something other than follow her precise eating routine. I followed the heartfelt study and tried to inspect the food that made me feel enlarged, exhausted, or cranky after eating them. I started with a vegetarian diet and, from then on, found the exact diet. Within four days, my dermatitis was gone - and now it really has stayed away forever.

The hardest part of the calming diet goes to cafes. It's amazing how regularly dairy sneaks into things! In any case, when you request vegetables, they fall under the spread. At least I appreciate cooking, so as far as I'm at home, I find the eating regimen extremely easy to follow. What I got from the book is that it's not about the amount of nutrition or the number of calories you devour. It's about whether food works for you. In case it causes aggravation, your histamines go up at that point, raising cortisol levels, meaning storing your fat forever, which can destroy your hormones and thyroid. It is this chain reaction caused by food that your exceptional body cannot tolerate. In any case, if you discover the food that you can handle, you can eat them. I never feel locked up.

It's annoying to design evening meals and consistently for yourself to cook, and it is becoming more expensive to buy consistently competitive products. But meat and dairy are also expensive, so I find that if I take those out, my spending on basic products remains about the same.

I have indeed shed pounds. However, the numbers that I notice more notably are the inches. I lost jitters from my stomach, and it's such a compliment because I never feel enlarged. I have more vitality, and I never feel that drowsiness after eating, or that grumpiness. Plus, my skin is finally incredible now, finally. I rarely come back.

Two years earlier, I was in pain. More than 25 years of tennis, despite general negligence for proper consideration and maintenance, had given me early joint inflammation and incessantly foggy cerebrum.

I was hopeless. Something had to change. The correct response was a strict selection of a soothing diet. The results were epic. I shed 24 pounds for six months. When sharing my story, the main question I got about the soothing diet is, "What are you eating?"

While the essential principles of the calming diet revolve around what not to eat (sugar, dairy, chicken, and prepared foods), building a dinner plan can be testing.

- **Before starting an anti-inflammatory diet** – If you're new to the smoothing diet, here are a couple interesting points:

- **Keep track of what you eat** – you will fight to be fertile in case you don't monitor your intake of fat, carbohydrates, and protein. Use the MyFitnessPal application. It is simple and free.

- **Moisturize** – Drink as much water as possible. That's all. You can have some lemon in it. Drinking water also prevents your body from generating a fake sense of hunger.

- **Stop eating late at night** – Give your body as much time as can be reasonably expected to process food before resting. Gut well-being is an immense piece of reducing aggravation.

- **Live by the 80/20 rule** – I still drink espresso and lager (both very sour), making sure they are within my 20 percent. Live 80 percent of your life, and you will feel gigantic.

- **Avoid anything sour** – Sour foods and drinks are the fallen angel. Enough said. This implies Coke Zero; you drink every day. Discard it.

- **Discover a routine** – The soothing diet is a lot easier if you can put it on a daily schedule. This applies to all eating regimens but also applies to this one.

- **Sun food Superfood Beet Powder** – As mentioned above, beets offer tremendous medical benefits, with nitrates being withheld as an elevator for athletic performance and blends to improve gut well-being, reduce circulation, and reduce aggravation.

These are the rules that worked for me. While your calming life can have different rules, I'm sure this is a good place to start.

Five times a week, I did not feel a decrease in the performance of whey to vegetable protein.

Chia seeds support the well-being of the heart and brain while at the same time providing a high content of omega-3 unsaturated fats, fiber, and protein, giving chia seeds a colossal calming diet.

The evening is when I will change my daily schedule because I am not a robot, I get desires and occasionally appreciate some change.

That said, there are two solid pieces that remain: significant hydration, and the second serving of alkalize greens.

The following is an overview of foods that I may use for dinner. One day I just choose one of these things, but I can flip them all consistently. In short, although they offer several benefits, they are interchangeable from my point of view.

Avocado

Avocados are an extraordinary source of healthy unsaturated fat and cancer prevention agents. Frankly, the calming properties of avocados are so strong that they can counterbalance less healthy dietary decisions.

Apple

Apples are high in normal cell fortifications and polyphenols.

Grain

Seventy-five percent of a cup of natural whole-grain cereal stirred oats with a hint of nectar and a few raspberries, blueberries, and blackberries. There is arguably no tremendous soothing benefit to grains. However, they are filled with fiber and tastes extraordinary.

Baked Food Organic Vegetables

Use a large part of a tablespoon of coconut oil and then add any natural vegetables you can get your hands on. We like to use:

- Broccoli

- Peas

- Spinach

- Garbanzo beans

- Onions

- Garlic

- Maize

- Brussels Sprouts

- Cauliflower

At that moment, we sprinkle Himalayan Sea salt and dark pepper. To give the dish some generosity, we include a prepared potato (we split a potato) or make natural red lentil pasta.

You can also go with berries or a large portion of an apple. For the nature of resting purposes, you should limit your food authorization to at least 600 hours.

Improvements: As far as supplements I take to help with exacerbation:

Turmeric and Onnit Krill Oil. I take both regularly and have effects that affected my joint pain.

The decisions you make in the market can affect the irritation in your body.

Anti-Inflammatory Diet Recipes to Help Your Immune System to Heal

Of course, inflammation is a process that helps white blood cells fight bacteria and viruses, but sometimes the inflammation persists and is known as chronic inflammation. Chronic inflammation can have various causes. Some doctors may suggest that it's because of irregular eating; others may suggest because of the lifestyle they chose. Chronic inflammation, if persistent, can affect and damage the immune system. Inflammation for that person can be recognized by heat or redness. In the event that a person can take medicine for his/her inflammation, and reduce the inflammation, the person can also weaken his/her immune system. So while saving the body, it can harm the body instead.

Certain steps can be taken to prevent or treat inflammation so that it has no effect on the immune system of the individual suffering from the disease. People who suffer from inflammation should follow a high fiber diet, including antioxidants and fatty acids, such as omega-three fatty acids. This suggests that the individual's diet should include content such as fruits, vegetables, fish, and vegetables.

A general diet can be made to improve the immune system. Some recipes are presented below:

Breakfast

Breakfast is the most important meal of the day, according to nutritionists. A healthy and satisfying breakfast is, therefore, a necessity. Some breakfast recipe suggestions may include:

- Berries (any kind) with oatmeal porridge

- Buckwheat along with seed porridge

- Scrambled eggs with turmeric

- Poached eggs, avocado, and salmon on bread

- Pineapple smoothie

Each of these recipes has its nutritional value and can be prepared every other day to maintain a healthy diet.

Berries With Oatmeal Porridge

This meal is not only rich in fiber and antioxidants but also in prebiotics. It is often suggested to take oats in steel instead of quick oats because they contain more fiber. Oats are a high fiber food; the type of fiber present in oats is called beta glycan. They are considered an important prebiotic for stomach bacteria, which help reduce the risk of obesity and inflammation.

Berries, especially blueberries, are high in antioxidants that prove to be very useful for anti-inflammatory purposes.

Ingredients

- Oats
- Gluten-free sliced oats (1 cup)
- Water (3 cups)
- Salt
- Dressing / Toppings
- Fresh/frozen treats like berries (to taste)
- Dry fruits (according to the preference of the person)
- Maple Syrup or whatever according to the consumer

Instructions

1 The usual ingredients are for four servings or according to the consumer's appetite.

2 Take the oats in a pan and start heating them. Then add

water and let it boil. The oats are getting thicker—Cook to the desired thickness. The oats are prepared. Consumers can now add sweets to their own tastes.

Buckwheat and Seed Porridge

It is often seen that people are sensitive to gluten eat oatmeal.

For people with gluten intolerance, buckwheat is a great alternative because it is gluten-free. Chia seeds consist of omega-three fatty acids, proteins, and fibers. Omega 3 fiber helps people fight inflammation along with a feeling of strength until the next meal.

In addition to a high nutritional value, it is an excellent basic breakfast.

The recipe is suitable for 6-8 people

Ingredients

- Buckwheat (1 cup)

- Oats (1/2 cup)

- Chia seeds (2 tablespoons)

- Milk (2 cups)

- Water (2 cups)

- Pear (1, grated with skin)

- Apple (1, grated with skin)

- Ginger (ground, 1 tsp)

- Cinnamon (ground, one teaspoon)

- Nutmeg (ground, 1/2 teaspoon)

- Cardamom (ground, 1/2 teaspoon)

- Nut butter (2 tablespoons)

- Vanilla extract (1 teaspoon)

- Honey (2 tablespoons)

For the Berry Compote

- Mixed frozen berries (500 g)

- Orange peel

- Caster sugar (1/3 cup)

- Corn flour (2 teaspoons)

- Water (1 tablespoon)

Instructions

1 Soak the oats and buckwheat overnight in cold water. Similarly, soak chia seeds in milk overnight in a separate bowl.

2 After soaking them overnight, drain the buckwheat and oats. Add them to the chia seeds and milk. Add all components in a frying pan with water, pear, and apple, all herbs, butter, honey, and vanilla. Cook all components until they form a smooth and creamy mixture. Keep adding water until the desired consistency is achieved. After serving, serve the porridge with your favorite toppings. The porridge can be premade and can be stored for up to 5 days.

3 To make the mixed berry compote, add the frozen

berries, juice, orange zest, and sugar in a saucepan and heat until boiling. Add cornflower to the bowl and mix until a smooth consistency is obtained. The berry compote can be served at room temperature

4 For the topping, the individual can choose yogurt or a frozen berry to taste.

__Turmeric and Scrambled Eggs__

Both components have their own nutritional value. Eggs are high in protein, while yolk has a high vitamin D content, which is known to reduce the effect of inflammation on the immune system. Furthermore, turmeric has a high content of cumin, a substance known for its oxidative properties that are beneficial in reducing inflammation.

The following recipe serves one

Ingredients

- Organic eggs (3)

- Turmeric (1 tsp)

- Chia Seeds (1 teaspoon)

- Organic coconut milk/cream (2 tablespoons)

- Salt

- Olive oil (2 teaspoons)

- Spinach leaves (100g)

- Super greens pesto (1 tablespoon)

Instructions

1 Add chia seeds, turmeric, egg, salt, coconut milk, and eggs in an arc. Beat the components and set aside. Add olive oil to a pan and let it heat up. Add spinach to the pan and fry for a while, then remove. Heat another pan and add olive oil to it. Then add the egg mixture to it.

Cook it until the eggs are creamy and add spinach to the mix. Serve the scrambled eggs with super green pesto.

Poached Eggs, Avocado, and Salmon on Bread

Avocado and salmon are high in omega-three fatty acids that help reduce inflammation. Fatty acids help the heart to stay healthy and save a person from heart disease. A person can also opt for a gluten-free alternative to bread, in case it is gluten intolerant.

Ingredients

- Bread (toasted, two slices)

- Avocado (broken, ½ cup)

- Lemon juice (1/4 teaspoon)

- Salt

- Pepper

- Smoked salmon (3.5 grams)

- Poached eggs (2)

- Spring onions (1 tablespoon)

- Microgreens

Instructions

1 Add the avocado to a small bowl and add lemon juice and salt. Mix all components and set aside. Poach the eggs and set them aside in an ice bath. Toast the bread while the eggs are cooked. Once toasted, add avocado and salmon to every slice of bread. Place the poached eggs on the toast. The individual can top with Kikkoman soy, microgreens, tomato, or bagel spices to suit the

individual.

Pineapple Smoothie

Pineapple consists of bromelain. Bromelain has significant properties that are beneficial for anti-inflammatory purposes. Further smoothies are high in fiber and have a firm feel.

Ingredients

- Kale (1 cup)
- Pineapple
- Banana
- Honey
- Peanut butter
- Greek yogurt
- Almond milk
- Ice cubes

Instructions

1 Add all components to a blender or juicer and mix them until they have a smooth consistency. To get a thicker consistency, also add ice cubes to the mix.

Lunch

The next meal of the day is lunch. Lunch should be hearty compared to breakfast. Some lunch recipes may be as follows:

- Hummus, grilled sauerkraut, and avocado sandwich

- Spinach and feta frittata

- Quinoa and lemon salad

- Lentils, beetroot, and hazelnut salad

- Cauliflower steak along with beans and tomatoes

- Lettuce wraps with smoked trout

Hummus, Grilled Sauerkraut, and Avocado Sandwich

This is the vegetarian alternative to Reuben used for an anti-inflammatory boost to an individual's mechanism. Sauerkraut consists of an important prebiotic that is important for the normal functioning of the stomach bacteria and the intestinal tract. The further grilled sandwich is low in sodium and calories compared to Reuben. In addition, hummus and avocado provide more useful nutrients compared to those found in meat used in Reuben.

Ingredients

- Pumpernickel bread (8 slices)
- Vegan butter
- Hummus (1 cup)
- Sauerkraut (1 cup)
- Avocado (1, peeled)

Instructions

1. Preheat the oven. Take eight slices of bread and spread on a baking tray, add butter to the slices. Add humus to half of the slices. Then add sauerkraut to the slices, to which hummus has already been added. Then add avocado over the same slices. Place the remaining four slices over the slices with avocado and the other components.

2. Bake these sandwiches for about 6-8 minutes. Keep turning the buns until browned and crispy on both sides.

Spinach and Feta Frittata

Green vegetables such as spinach are high in important polyphenols such as quercetin and coenzyme Q10, which are considered integral inflammatory remedies. Coenzyme Q10 is responsible for reducing inflammation; it also helps the patient against other diseases such as diabetes.

The ingredients can contain four servings with 153 calories per serving.

Ingredients

- Olive oil (1 teaspoon)

- Brown onion (1/2, sliced)

- Garlic (1 teaspoon)

- Spinach (250 g)

- Eggs (4)

- Crumbled feta cheese (1/2 cup)

- Salt

- Pepper

Instructions

1. Preheat the grill. Heat the oil on a non-stick pan. Cook the onion and spinach on the oil until the onion turns brown. Fry the spinach with oil. Remove both components and allow them to cool. Beat the eggs in a bowl, add the spinach, onion, feta to the mixture. Add

salt and pepper to taste. Bake the eggs and let the frittata turn. Place the pan in the grill until the frittata is golden brown and crispy. Turn the frittata and egg over on the plate and serve with a salad.

Quinoa and Lemon Salad

This dish is great for people with gluten intolerance and those following a vegan diet. Quinoa has a high amount of protein and other important nutrients, and citrus fruits also have many components that have antioxidant properties. Vitamin C is also very beneficial for people who suffer from inflammation.

Ingredients

- Cooked Quinoa (1 cup)

- Oranges (2)

- Celery Rib (1)

- Brazil nuts (minced meat, 20 g)

- Green onion (1)

- Parsley (chopped, ¼ cup)

- For the toppings

- Orange juice

- Lemon juice (1/2 teaspoon)

- Ginger (grated, 1/2 teaspoon)

- Vinegar (1 tsp)

- Garlic (1 small clove)

- Salt

- Black pepper

- Cinnamon

Instructions

1   Cut all oranges and squeeze juice without wasting anything. Add the juice with the remaining dressing ingredients to a food processor and mix until smooth. Cut the remaining oranges in a bowl.

2   Add the remaining ingredients and mix. Bring all the components together and serve.

3   Choose Quinoa that is gluten-free.

Lentils, Beetroot, and Hazelnut Salad

Lentils are rich in protein and very useful for people on a vegan diet. According to a nutritionist, lentils and beetroot are high in fiber, protein, and vitamin E. Vitamin E also acts as an antioxidant.

Furthermore, Beetroot contains Betaine, which serves as an anti-inflammatory agent.

The ingredient is suitable for 2-3 people.

Ingredients

- Salad

- Lentils (1 cup)

- Water (2 cups)

- Salt

- Beetroot (boiled, 3)

- Spring onions (sliced, 2)

- Hazelnuts (2 tablespoons)

- Coin

- Parsley

- Ginger dressing

- Fresh ginger (3/4 inch)

- Olive oil (6 tablespoons)

- Dijon Mustard (1 tablespoon.)

- Apple cider vinegar (1 tablespoon.)

- Salt

- Pepper

Instructions

1 Cut the beetroot into small cubes. Put the lentils in a pan with water, cover the pan and let the liquid evaporate, so that the lentils become mushy, that is, let the lentils boil for about 15-20 minutes. After cooking, put the lentils in a bowl and let them cool, then add beetroot, hazelnuts, spices, onions, and mix everything.

2 To make the ginger dressing, add ginger, oil, mustard, and vinegar in a food processor and mix until smooth. Finally, add the dressing to the salad, and it is ready to serve.

Cauliflower Steak Along With Beans and Tomatoes

Cauliflower is high in fiber and antioxidants. It can also prove to be an inflammatory agent and a prebiotic for the stomach bacteria.

The following can serve two people, with 1141 calories per serving.

Ingredients

- Cauliflower (2 pounds)

- Olive oil (1/2 cup)

- Kosher salt (2 teaspoons)

- Black pepper (1 tsp)

- Green beans (8 ounces)

- Garlic cloves (minced, 3)

- Lemon zest (3/4 teaspoon)

- Parsley (chopped, 1/3 cup)

- Panko (1/3 cup)

- Parmesan cheese (1/4 cup)

- White beans (15 grams)

- Red cherry tomato (1 cup / 6 ounce)

- Mayonnaise (3 tablespoons)

- Dijon mustard (1 teaspoon).

Instructions

1   Preheat the oven. Cut the cauliflower so that a kind of steak is created. Remnants can be used afterward. Place the cauliflower on a baking tray. Brush both sides of the cauliflower with salt, pepper, and oil and cook until the cauliflower turns brown. This takes about 30 minutes.

2   Add oil, salt, and pepper to the green beans and cook until the beans are blistered. This takes about 15 minutes.

3   Now add garlic, zest, parsley, salt, pepper, and remaining oil to the boil and mix. Add panko and parmesan to the bowl and mix. Then add beans and tomatoes to the mixture—mix mayonnaise and mustard in a separate bowl. Remove the beans and cauliflower from the oven. Divide the mayonnaise mixture over the cooked cauliflower. Then add the panko mixture. Add beans and cook until the beans are crispy.

4   Cut the cauliflower and divide it among the vegetables.

Lettuce Wraps With Smoked Trout

Trout, compared to other fish, is considered an oily fish with a high content of omega-three fatty acids. Furthermore, it is a great option for people with gluten intolerance.

The recipe provides four servings with 423 calories per serving.

Ingredients

- Carrots (2)

- Cucumber (1/2)

- Shallots (sliced, ½ cup)

- Jalapeño peppers with seeds (sliced, 1/4 cup)

- Lime juice (2 tablespoons)

- Sugar (1 tablespoon)

- Fish sauce (1 tablespoon)

- Smoked trout (skinless, 2 cups, 9 ounces)

- Tomatoes (1 cup)

- Mint leaves (1/2 cup)

- Basil leaves (1/2 cup)

- Romaine lettuce (16 small)

- Asian sweet chili sauce (1/3 cup)

- Roasted peanuts (1/4 cup)

Instructions

1 Cut the carrots and cucumbers lengthwise and then into wedges and place them in a bowl. Then add shallots, chilies, lime juice, sugar, and fish sauce to the mixture and let the marinating rest.

2 Add trout and tomatoes to the vegetables in the bowl and mix. Then drain the trout and add basil and mint to the mixture. Arrange the lettuce on a platter. Add the trout and the vegetable mixture to the dish. Add the salad and top with peanuts.

Supper

Dinner is the last meal of the day. After an exhausting day, one often wants to eat something savory. The following are some hearty dishes that a person seeking an anti-inflammatory diet is looking for.

- Salmon with zucchini pasta and pesto

- Roasted cauliflower, fennel, and ginger soup

- Lentil and chicken soup and sweet potato

- Salmon with greens and cauliflower rice

- Shrimps and vegetable curry

Salmon with Zucchini Pasta and Pesto

Zucchini is a great alternative when it comes to considering gluten intolerance. Salmon is also rich in omega-3 fatty acids, an essential part of the diet of an inflammatory patient.

Ingredients

- Salmon steaks (2)

- Zucchini (1)

- Avocado (1)

- Parmesan cheese (grated, 1/4 cup)

- Pesto (1 tablespoon)

- Lemon (half)

- Black pepper

Instructions

1. Season the salmon with lemon juice, pepper, and any flavor to taste and cook it. The next step is to make zucchini noodles (cut the zucchini lengthwise with a knife). Add avocado, lemon juice, pepper, and pesto and mash them all together.

2. Add the cooked salmon to a bowl of avocado puree and zucchini noodles. When serving, add pesto o parmesan according to the person's taste.

Roasted Cauliflower, Fennel, and Ginger Soup

Anti-inflammatory y diets should include a high vegetable intake as vegetables are high in fiber and other nutrients. Thick soups like this are a great source of increasing the patient's intake of vegetables.

Ingredients

- Red onion (1)
- Garlic cloves (4)
- Cauliflower (1/2)
- Fennel bulbs (2)
- Each stock (500 g)
- Hummus (3 tablespoons)
- Turmeric (1 tsp.)
- Cinnamon
- Black pepper
- Sage leaves (1 teaspoon)
- Fennel seed (pinch)
- Wheat-free Tamari (2 tablespoons)
- Lemon (2 tablespoons)
- Ginger (1)

Instructions

1   Prepare the Golden Gut Blend by mixing one teaspoon of turmeric with a small pinch of black pepper and cinnamon. Preheat the oven. Take a baking tray and add onion, garlic, cauliflower, and fennel. Fry the vegetables until crispy. This takes about 30-35 minutes.

2   Remove the vegetables from the oven and put them in the blender and mix until creamy. Put the vegetables in a pan and heat. The individual can season to add flavor as desired by the individual. The soup can be served warm.

Lentil and Chicken Soup and Sweet Potato

Sweet potatoes are high in minerals and nutrients such as vitamins A, B, and C. They also have beneficial factors that can act as antioxidants such as calcium and iron. Lentils are also a source of fiber and protein.

Ingredients

- Chicken carcass (cooked, 1)

- Sweet Potatoes (2)

- Lentils (3/4 cup)

- Salt (1 teaspoon)

- Extra virgin olive oil (2 tablespoons)

- Celery sticks (10)

- Garlic cloves (slices, 6)

- Grated chicken (1½ cups)

- Escarole (1/2)

- Chopped dill (1/2 cup)

- Lemon juice (2 tablespoons)

Instructions

1 Add chicken carcass, potatoes, lentils, and salt to a saucepan, with 8 cups of water, and cook until the vegetables are tender. After cooking, discard the chicken carcass from the mixture.

2   Add celery and garlic and oil and cook until both are browned. This takes about 12 minutes. Now add the celery, garlic, grated chicken and escarole to the soup and cook for about 5 minutes. Remove the mixture from the heat. Add lemon juice and dill while serving.

Salmon With Greens and Cauliflower Rice

Cauliflower rice is high in nutrients and high in fiber. They also contain a high amount of antioxidants and fiber.

Ingredients

- Salmon fillet (2)

- Brussels sprouts (10-12)

- Kale

- Cauliflower Rice

- Olive/coconut oil (3 tablespoons)

- Curry powder (1 tsp)

- Salt

To make the marinade:

- Tamari sauce (1/4 cup)

- Dijon Mustard (1 teaspoon)

- Sesame oil (1 teaspoon)

- Honey/maple syrup (1 tsp)

- Sesame seeds (1 tablespoon)

Instructions

1. Preheat the oven. Add sprouts with herbs to a baking sheet and roast for about 20 minutes. Combine all remaining ingredients in a large bowl and beat. Remove

the Brussels sprouts and add salmon to them. Pour the marinade and cook the salmon again for 13 to 15 minutes. Add kale and oil to the pan and sauté.

2   Add cauliflower to a separate bowl and season with curry powder and salt. Fry them separately in a pan. Finally, add all the individual components, namely salmon, Brussels sprouts, cauliflower, and kale and serve.

Shrimps and Vegetable Curry

A shrimp contains astaxanthin, which is beneficial for its anti-inflammatory properties. Carrots and other vegetables have polyphenol content and have similar properties.

Ingredients

- Butter/coconut oil (3 tablespoons)

- Onions (chopped, 1)

- Coconut milk (1 cup)

- Curry powder (3 teaspoons)

- Shrimp (1 pound)

- Cauliflower or vegetable of your choice (1 bag)

Instructions

1 Add oil to a pan and add the onion. Fry the onions until brown and soft. Once the onions are soft, add coconut milk, curry spices, and other spices to the mix to your taste.

2 Cook so that the flavors are incorporated into the mix. Steam the vegetables. Remove tails from shrimp. Add the shrimps and cook until the shrimps are soft and cooked. Serve the prawns with the steamed vegetables with butter and salad. The individual can determine the dressing of his choice.

All of the listed dishes are nutrient-rich and recommended by a nutritionist to include in their anti-inflammatory diet. All these recipes are made from elements with a lot of fiber, fatty acids, and other nutrients needed are to preserve inflammation.

Anti-Inflammatory Diet Recipes From Preventing Disease

Inflammation can put you at risk for cardiovascular disease. Furthermore, it can also lead to strokes or obesity. All these diseases may not be decisive because of inflammation but persist due to inflation. Some recipes that can help an individual fight or control inflammation are:

1   Citrus salad with yogurt

2   Pan-seared salmon

3   Grilled salmon with orange spice sauce

4   Carrots and Brussels sprouts

5   Curried chicken salad with spiced chickpeas and raita.

A common trait that can be seen in all dishes is that all dishes are high in nutrients. Fish made up of omega-three fatty acids are also included in most recipes suggested for anti-inflammatory agents.

Citrus Salad With Yogurt

The recipe makes six servings, and per serving is 287 calories.

Ingredients

- Pink grapefruit (1)

- Tangerines/Minneolas (2 large)

- Oranges (3)

- Dried cranberries (half a cup)

- Honey (2 tablespoons)

- Ground Cinnamon (1/4 tablespoon)

- Ginger (chopped, 2/3 cup)

- Brown sugar (1/4 cup)

- Dried cranberries

- Greek yogurt

(Greek yogurt is a luxury meal and hard to find in local markets. However, it can be prepared at home. Take plain yogurt and add it to a jar of cheesecloth. Leave it overnight).

Instructions

1. Divide the grapefruit and tangerines in half and the third, respectively. Put them in a bowl with all the juices. Slice the oranges and put them in the bowl. Add honey and cinnamon to dried cranberries.

2. Add yogurt and ginger separately and refrigerate. You

can enjoy the yogurt later with a topping of fruit and brown sugar.

Pan-Seared Salmon Salad

Two servings (390 calories per serving).

Ingredients

- Salmon fillets (2)

- Lemon juice (1 ½ tablespoon)

- Olive oil (1 ½ tablespoon)

- Salt

- Pepper

- Baby arugula leaves (3 cups)

- Grape or cherry tomatoes (2/3 cups)

- Red onion (1/4 cup)

- Vinegar (1 tablespoon)

Instructions

1 Add salmon fish in a bowl, then add lemon, olive oil, salt, and pepper and let it rest. Cook the salmon on a nonstick surface and toss on both sides to continue cooking. The skin should remain crispy.

2 While preparing the salmon, add some arugula leaves to a bowl of tomatoes and onion. Finally, before serving, add salt and pepper with vinegar.

Grilled Salmon With Orange Spice Sauce

The necessary ingredients are sufficient for six servings, each serving to count only 197 calories.

Ingredients

- Orange (1)

- Onion (thinly sliced, 1)

- Olive oil (1 ½ tablespoon)

- Salmon fillet (6 ounces)

- Chopped fresh dill (3 tablespoons)

- Orange juice (1/2 cup)

- Green onions (sliced, 1/4 cup)

- Lemon juice (1 ½ tablespoon)

Instructions

1. Preheat the oven. Add the orange slices, cover with oil and onion, and cook until the onion is brown. Now place the salmon in the center of the dish and add salt, pepper, and dill. Roast the salmon for about 8 minutes. Mix all remaining components, such as orange and lemon juice, dill, and green onions in a bowl.

2. Place the salmon on a plate with the onion and orange slices. Pour the sauce over the salmon and finish the look by garnishing with the remaining orange slices.

Carrots and Brussels Sprouts

The ingredients can be used to make six servings, and each serving has about 150 calories.

Ingredients

- Chopped shallot (2 tablespoons)

- Unsalted butter (3 tablespoons)

- Carrots (1 pound)

- Brussels sprouts (1 pound)

- Water (1/3 cup)

- Cider vinegar (1 tablespoon)

Instructions

1. Cut the carrots into diagonal pieces and the sprouts in half. Add the shallot to a skillet over medium heat and cook until the shallots are soft. Then add Brussels sprouts, carrots, salt and pepper, and cook until the vegetable brown.

2. Then add water and cook for about 8 minutes, until the vegetables are soft. Stir with vinegar, salt, and pepper to flavor the mixture. Occasionally, the vegetables can be pre-cut for convenience.

Curried Chicken Salad With Spiced Chickpeas and Raita

The ingredients are enough to make four servings with 635 calories per serving.

Ingredients

Curried Chicken Salad

- Onion (chopped, 1 cup)

- Garlic (minced, one tablespoon)

- Ginger (chopped. 1 tablespoon)

- Vegetable oil (2 tablespoons)

- Curry powder (1 tablespoon)

- Cumin (1 tablespoon)

- Tomatoes (chopped, 1 cup)

- Plain yogurt (1 cup)

- Cilantro (2 tablespoons)

- Rotisserie chicken (1, 3-4 cups)

- Red grapes (1 cup)

Chickpeas

- Vegetable oil (1 tablespoon)

- Chickpeas (dried, 19 grams)

- Cumin (1 tsp)

- Turmeric (1/2 teaspoon)

- Cayenne (1/4 teaspoon)

Raita

- Yogurt (1 cup)

- Cucumber (chopped, peeled and seedless)

- Mint (minced meat, two tablespoons)

- Almonds (toasted, ½ cup)

Instructions

1   Prepare Curried Chicken Salad adding garlic, ginger, and onion to oil in a pan and heat them slowly by occasionally stirring until soft. After the onion has browned, add curry, cumin, and salt and cook for two more minutes.

2   Then add tomatoes to the mixture until a sauce forms for about 5 minutes. Add it to a bowl of yogurt, chicken, and cilantro. Stir all components and let them rest at room temperature.

3   Put the chickpeas in a saucepan, cook the chickpeas in oil until it simmers. Then add cumin, turmeric, salt, and cayenne pepper and cook. Let them cool to room temperature.

4   For the raita, add yogurt, chopped cucumber, mint, and salt in a pot and stir to combine.

5   Finally, add the curries chicken, raita, and chickpeas in a pot, ready to serve. For convenience, all components can

be stored independently one day in advance and reused later. However, after mixing, the food remains good for about 6 hours.

Top 50 Anti-Inflammatory Foods

Vegetables

1　Broccoli

2　Spinach

3　Rosemary

4　Tomatoes

5　Cocoa

6　Mushrooms

7　Beets

8　Kale

9　Collard

10　Sweet potatoes

Fatty Fish

1　Salmon

2　Herring

3　Mackerels

4　Sardines

5　Oyster

6　Anchovies

Cereals

1　Khorasan wheat

2   Chia seeds

3   Raw oats

4   Black beans

5   Millet

6   Barley

7   Brown rice

8   Chickpeas

Fruits

1   Strawberries

2   Red berries

3   Blueberries

4   Raspberries

5   Blackberries

6   Avocadoes

7   Grapes

8   Cherries

9   Pineapple

10   Apples

11   Oranges

12   Bell peppers

13   Chili peppers

Spices

1   Turmeric

2   Ginger

3   Garlic

4   Cinnamon

5   Cayenne

6   Black pepper

7   Clove

Others

1   Coconut oil

2   Raw honey

3   Extra virgin olive oil

4   Green tea

5   Chocolate

6   Nuts

Meal Plan With a Shopping List

Day 1

Breakfast	Lunch	Dinner
Blueberry-banana overnight oats	**Green salad with Edamame and beets**	**Walnut-rosemary with salmon**
Shopping list	**Shopping list**	**Shopping list**
Coconut oil beverage	Salad greens	Dijon mustard
Oat	Edamame	Garlic
Chia seed	Beet	Lemon
Banana	Red wine vinegar	Rosemary
Blueberries	Cilantro and pepper	Honey and pepper
Maple syrup	Extra virgin olive oil	Salmon fillets, walnut, Olive oil and breadcrumbs

Day 2

Breakfast	Lunch	Dinner
Raspberries-kefir power smoothie	**Vegan supper food Buddha bowl**	**Indian spiced cauliflower and chickpea salad**
Shopping list	**Shopping list**	**Shopping list**
Banana	Quinoa	Curry powder and olive oil
Raspberries	Lemon	Cauliflower and garbanzo bean
Kefir	Hummus and edamame	Carrot, yogurt and lime juice
Peanut	Baby kale and baby beet	Pepper, ginger and jalapeno chili pepper
Flax meal	Avocadoes and sunflower seed	Lettuce, milk and red onion

Day 3

Breakfast	Lunch	Dinner
	Vegan supper food Buddha bowl	**Salmon with creamy garlic dressing**
Shopping list	**Shopping list**	**Shopping list**
Blueberries	Quinoa	Salmon fillets
Yogurt	Lemon	Yogurt and mayonnaise
Walnut	Hummus and edamame	Lemon juice and parmesan cheese
Green tea	Baby kale and baby beet	Garlic, pepper, and chives
	Avocadoes and sunflower seed	Soy sauce, kale, and broccoli
		Red cabbage and sunflower seed

Day 4

Breakfast	Lunch	Dinner
Cocoa-chia pudding with raspberries	**Green salad with Edamame and beets**	**Sweet potatoes with hummus dressings**
Shopping list	**Shopping list**	**Shopping list**
Almond milk	Salad greens	Potatoes
Chia seed	Edamame	Kale
Maple syrup	Beet	Black beans
Cocoa powder	Red wine vinegar	Hummus
Vanilla	Cilantro and pepper	Water
Raspberries	Extra virgin olive oil	
Almonds		

Day 5

Breakfast	Lunch	Dinner
Raspberries-kefir power smoothie	**Turmeric-ginger tahini dip**	**Korean steak kimchi and cauliflower rice bowls**
Shopping list	**Shopping list**	**Shopping list**
Banana	Ginger	Eggs
Raspberries	Turmeric	Sesame oil
Kefir	Tahini	Cauliflower
Peanut butter	Garlic	Scallions
Flax meal	Rice vinegar	Sirloin steak
		Ginger
		Gochujang and sesame seed
		Carrots and kimchi

Day 6

Breakfast	Lunch	Dinner
Cocoa-chia pudding with raspberries	**Green salad with Edamame and beets**	**Hummus crusted chicken**
Shopping list	**Shopping list**	**Shopping list**
Almond milk	Salad greens	Hummus
Chia seed	Edamame	Cumin
Maple syrup	Beet	Limon
Cocoa powder	Red wine vinegar	Paprika
Vanilla	cilantro and pepper	Chicken breasts
Raspberries	Extra virgin olive oil	Sesame
Almonds		Parsley

Day 7

Breakfast	Lunch	Dinner
Turmeric latte	**Avocadoes egg salad sandwich**	**One-pot garlicky shrimp and spinach**
Shopping list	**Shopping list**	Shopping list
Honey	Avocadoes	Olive oil
Turmeric	Lemon	Garlic
Almond milk	Avocadoes oil	Spinach
Ginger	Chives	Lemon
Pepper	Celery	Shrimp
cinnamon	Egg and bread	Pepper
	Pepper and lettuce	Parsley

Two Weeks Meal Plan for an Anti-Inflammatory Diet

Anti-Inflammatory Diet Recipes for Easy Weight Loss

Inflammation is a condition in which the body's white blood cells protect the body's immune system against viruses and other bacteria. However, in some cases, this can be disadvantageous. Therefore, many nutritionists recommend an anti-inflammatory diet to deal with the condition.

An anti-inflammatory diet includes foods that many nutritionists recommend as part of a clean and healthy meal. Some anti-inflammatory foods recommended for a diet may include fruits and vegetables, foods rich in fiber such as whole grains, beans, fish, herbs, and spices.

However, it is recommended to avoid processed and fatty foods. It is further advised to avoid foods with high sugar or fat content. Furthermore, fast food, coffee, and similar items should be avoided by people who suffer from inflammation.

Do's and Don'ts of an Anti-Inflammatory Diet

Do

The diet should include **fruits and vegetables**. The individual is advised to take vegetables with high vitamin K content, such as spinach, broccoli, cabbage, and kale. The vegetables are known to fight inflammation. Further fruits such as raspberries, blackberries, and cherries should be added to the individual diet. These fruits tend to have a pigment necessary for their color that helps patients with inflammation.

The diet should include **fiber-rich** foods, as fiber helps patients suffering from inflammation. For this purpose, whole grains such as brown rice and oatmeal can be added to the individual's diet.

Since beans with high fiber content can be included in the person's diet, beans not only process high fiber but also contain antioxidants that are useful for people with inflammation.

Fish should also be included in an anti-inflammatory diet because fish contains omega-three fatty acids, which helps fight inflammation. According to some nutritionists, fish should be eaten at least twice a week. Some suggested fish are salmon and sardines etc.

The last thing to add to an anti-inflammatory diet is **spices** like turmeric and spices. Herbs and spices are known to contain a rich amount of antioxidants that help people with inflammation.

Don't

Some of the things that are advised to be avoided by people with inflammation are:

Anything with **high sugar content** should also be avoided by people who suffer from inflammation. This is because foods with high sugar content can be easily consumed, leading to diseases such as high blood sugar, obesity, or even high cholesterol, all of which lead to inflammatory diseases. A nutritionist often advises removing all that food, including sodas, sugary drinks, and even honey, from the diet of inflammatory patients.

Foods with **saturated fats,** such as processed foods, should be avoided.

Dairy products such as butter and cheese, if consumed lightly, have no significant effect. However, if consumed in large amounts, they are likely to cause inflammation due to the saturated fat it contains.

Fried foods also cause inflammation. The thing to note here is that frying food in vegetable oil doesn't make it healthy because it increases the omega 6s content rather than the omega 3s. This is not recommended in inflammatory patients.

Trans fats that can be labeled with partially hydrogenated oils on most coffee milk or margarine is also a major cause of the high cholesterol, causing inflammation. Trans fat is one of the most dangerous food products consumed by inflammatory patients, so patients should avoid even small amounts of the substance.

After discussing the main content of what should and should not be added to an inflammatory patient's diet, a 14-day meal plan can be drawn up. The diet plan focuses on clean eating and leads the patient to consume an estimated 1,200 calories each day for healthy functioning. The consumer can increase the number of calories by increasing the content of the individual foods on the list. The diet or consumption of calories may vary from person to person, depending on the individual's effort during the day.

Week 1

Day 1

Breakfast

Breakfast consists of a serving of raspberries with muesli. What you should pay attention to when buying mussel is that the consumer should choose a brand that has less added sugars in the muesli. This meal contains about 267 calories for the day.

Morning snack

The consumer is advised to take pure orange juice or have an orange. This meal contains about 62 calories for the day.

Lunch

Lunch is one of the basic meals of the day. To have a healthy yet reasonable lunch, the patient should take about two servings of beans (preferably white) with a vegetable salad. Lunch is rich in nutrients, antioxidants, and fiber and contains about 360 calories for the day.

Evening snack

Just like the morning snack, the consumer can take apple juice (unprocessed and homemade) or a simple apple. The estimated calorie for this meal is 95 calories.

Supper

Like lunch, dinner is also one of the basic meals of the day. Consumers are advised to eat almost two servings of kale salad with beets and wild rice. The consumer can eat brown or wild rice. The meal also consists of a portion of Balsamic Dijon Chicken. The meal contains about 420 calories for the day.

Day 2

Breakfast

The consumer is advised to take one serving of avocado on an egg. It is easy to prepare. It is also rich in nutrients and low in calories. Breakfast is 270 calories a day.

Doctors also recommend looking for sauces with less added sugar in their ingredients.

Morning snack

Fruits and vegetables are the keys to healthy eating. As on the first day, the consumer is advised to eat a pear. Together with its nutrition facts, it is only 101 calories per day.

Lunch

Lunch for the second day consists of vegetables. It is advised to use fresh vegetables instead of stored vegetables.

Lunch consists of:

- Salad (2 cups green)
- Cucumber
- Balsamic-Dijon Chicken (Half Breast)
- Lemon-Tahini (2 tablespoons as a dressing)
- Sunflower seeds

Balsamic-Dijon Chicken

This recipe is free of oils, sugar, and other processed foods. The following recipe is suitable for four people.

Ingredients

- Boneless chicken breast (4, i.e., 1 pound)

- Dijon mustard (a third cup)

- Balsamic vinegar (3 tablespoons)

- Garlic (2 cloves, chopped)

- Thyme / Basil (2 tablespoons)

Instructions

1 Take the required amount of chicken and set aside. Then prepare the marinade. Take mustard, balsamic, thyme, and garlic and stir them in a bowl.

2 Add the marinade with chicken and refrigerate for 5-12 hours. Keep turning the sides. While cooking, place the chicken on the grill, and cook as desired by the consumer. Bake for 6-7 minutes and continue brushing the remaining marinade on the chicken for those seven minutes.

Lemon –Tahini

Ingredients

- Lemon juice (3 tablespoons)

- Water (2 tablespoons)

- Tahini (2 tablespoons)

- Garlic (1 clove, chopped)

- Salt

- Cayenne pepper

Instructions

1. Take all listed ingredients in a bowl and mix together to make a healthy and fun dressing.

Evening snack

The consumer is advised to take an orange. It contains about 62 calories a day.

Supper

The individual can take a single serving of pumpkin and red lentil curry, along with half a bowl of brown rice.

Pumpkin and Red Lentil Curry

The dish is not only rich in nutrients; but also in flavor, which complements the complexity of the dish.

The following serves five and can be eaten with naan or rice.

Ingredients

- Canola oil (2 tablespoons)

- Onion (diced, half cup)

- Garlic (minced)

- Curry powder/garam masala (2 tablespoons)

- Butternut squash

- Red lentils (1 cup)

- Tomatoes (chopped, 1 cup)

- Salt

- Water (4 cups)

- Coconut milk (1-14 grams)

- Lime wedges (5)

- Coriander for garnish

Instructions

1   Heat the oil. Add ginger, curry powder and garlic and cook until the onions are warm. Then add the remaining ingredients, i.e., lentils, pumpkin, salt, pepper and tomato, and cook.

2   Add water to the mixture and cover and cook until all components have broken down and mixed into one mixture. Finally, add coconut milk and cook it. Serve delicious curry with cilantro or lime wedges.

Day 3

Breakfast

Take Muesli together with raspberries for breakfast for the day. Take just one serving that makes up about 287 calories of the meal.

Morning snack

Keeping snacks fresh and oil-free is key to eating clean. Take a medium-sized orange, which makes up about 62 calories a day.

Lunch

Take squash and red lentil curry. This meal contains about 326 calories for the day.

Evening snack

Dry fruit is also an important part of a healthy diet. Take about 12 almonds as an evening snack, which equates to about 92 calories for the day.

Supper

For dinner, take brown rice (1 cup) along with a single serving of Asian Tilapia with stir-fried green beans.

Asian Tilapia With Stir-Fried Green Beans

Ingredients

The ingredients are for four servings:

- Fresh/frozen tilapia fillets (4-5 Ounce)

- Soy sauce (1/4 cup)

- Fresh ginger (grated, one tablespoon)

- Sesame oil (toasted, one tablespoon)

- Garlic (minced, one clove)

- Water (1/4 cup)

- Green beans (1 pound)

- Canola oil (1 tablespoon)

- Nonstick spray

- Sesame seeds (toasted, one tablespoon)

- Sliced Green Onions

Instructions

1. Wash the fish and store it in a baking dish. Mix the soy sauce, ginger, sesame oil, and garlic to make the marinade. Add the marinade to the dish and cover with foil. Let the fish rest for 20 minutes. While the fish is set to a non-stick pan, add beans and water and heat them.

2. Add canola oil to the beans and let them get crispy. Add

the spray to another nonstick pan and place the fish on it for 6-8 minutes. Add sesame seeds while cooking. Add the fish, beans, and the remaining marinade to a bowl, and it is easy to serve.

Day 4

Breakfast

Boil half a cup of oats in milk. Take them with a medium chopped plum. This breakfast contains approximately 257 calories.

Morning snack

Take an apple; it consists of 95 unprocessed calories.

Lunch

Have a serving of sandwiches with vegetables and hummus. The consumer is advised to check whether the hummus has added sugars and, in that case, avoid the hummus.

Sandwich With Vegetables and Hummus

It is a hearty lunch with a fresh and satisfying feeling.

Ingredients

- Bread (2 slices)

- Hummus (3 tablespoons)

- Avocado (mash)

- Salad greens (half cup)

- Red bell pepper (1/2, sliced)

- Cucumber

- Grated Carrot (1/4 cup)

Instructions

1 Take the bread slices. Cover one slice with hummus and the other slice with avocado puree. Fill the sandwich with vegetables such as cucumber, carrot, etc.

2 Finally, cut the prepared sandwich in half, and it is ready to serve.

Evening snack

The consumer can take a banana or banana shake. Whatever the consumer finds satisfying.

Supper

The consumer is advised to eat one serving of chicken with Brussels sprouts. The dish contains 432 calories for the day.

Chicken with Brussel Sprouts

Ingredients

- Sweet potatoes (1 pound; cut into wedges)

- Extra virgin olive oil (2 tablespoons)

- Salt

- Pepper

- Brussels sprouts (4 cups, quartered)

- Cumin (grounded; ½ tablespoon)

- Thyme (dried 1/2 tablespoon)

- Sherry vinegar (3 tablespoons)

- Boneless chicken thigh (1 ¼ pound)

Instructions

1. Preheat the oven.

2. Toss the sweet potato with oil, salt, and pepper on a baking sheet and roast for 15 minutes. Add Brussels sprouts and do the same. Take the chicken and add cumin, salt, pear, and thyme. Roast the chicken until completely cooked. Serve the dish with the vegetables.

Day 5

Breakfast

For this meal, serve the consumer with Peanut Butter Banana Cinnamon Toast. The consumer can use bread (gluten-free) to their own taste. The meal is 290 calories. Furthermore, when choosing peanut butter, it is advised to choose a brand without added sugars.

Morning snack

The consumer can take half a cup of raspberries. The snack contains 32 calories for the day.

Lunch

The consumer can get almost 4 cups of white beans and vegetable salad. It is a hearty meal and contains 360 calories per day.

Supper

Because the consumer misses the evening snack, he can opt for a hearty dinner. The scheduled dinner is 543 calories for the day. Consumers are advised to take one serving of mutton cutlets with Garlicky Broccoli.

Day 6

Breakfast

For this meal, the consumer can take about half a cup of oatmeal and take it with milk. Furthermore, the consumer can take a chopped plum. This is approximately 257 calories.

Morning snack

Just like the past few days, a snack is often light. The consumer is advised to take a pear or another fruit. This is approximately 101 calories per day.

Lunch

The consumer can enjoy a sandwich with vegetables and hummus during lunch. The recipe is shared above.

Evening snack

By keeping the snacks light, the individual is advised to take an orange or other similar fruit.

Supper

For dinner, the person should eat a single serving of cauliflower rice filled with pepper. Furthermore, the individual can enjoy a salad mixed with Vinaigrette Citrus. Recipes for both dishes are shared below.

Cauliflower Rice-Stuffed Pepper

Cauliflower is a sturdy alternative to the traditional bell pepper filling.

Ingredients

The following recipe serves four

- Bell pepper (4)

- Cauliflower florets (2 cups)

- Olive oil (2 tablespoons)

- Salt

- Ground pepper

- Chopped onion (half cup)

- Minced meat (1 pound)

- Garlic (minced, two cloves)

- Dried Oregano (1/2 tablespoon)

- Tomato sauce (without salt)

- Mozzarella (half cup shredded)

Instructions

1. Cut the peppers into slices. Remove excess substance from the pepper. Cook the bell pepper until soft, then set aside.

2. Boil the cauliflower until broken. Put one tablespoon of

oil in a pan and add cauliflower rice and salt and pepper and cook until the rice has browned. Add the mixture to a bowl. Then add the remaining oil, pepper, and onion in the pan and cook for about 3-4 minutes. Then add beef, garlic, oregano, the remaining salt, and pepper.

3. Cook the mixture until the beef has broken down and is no longer pink, then add cauliflower rice and mix. Finally, take the peppers in an oven dish and add a good amount of the mixture together with cheese. Heat/cook the peppers in the preheated oven and serve.

Vinaigrette Citrus

Ingredients

The following ingredients prepare the dish sufficiently for eight servings.

- Shallot (quartered)

- Orange zest (1 tablespoon)

- Orange juice (1/4 cup)

- Lemon juice (2 tablespoons)

- Dijon mustard (2 tablespoons)

- Salt

- Ground pepper

- Olive oil (¼ cup)

- Organic rapeseed oil/avocado oil (1/4 cup)

Instructions

1. Add all ingredients to the food processor and run until smooth contents are obtained. The contents can be cooled for further use.

Day 7

Breakfast

The individual is advised to drink two cups of avocado green smoothie. It contains about 307 calories for the day.

Avocado Green Smoothie

The recipe is suitable for two people.

Ingredients

- Coconut milk/almond milk (1 ¼ cup)

- Avocado (1)

- Banana (1)

- Apple (1)

- Celery (chopped)

- Kale leaves/spinach (2 cups)

- Ginger (1 inch)

- Ice cubes (8)

Instructions

1. Add all the contents to the blender and mix until the mixture is smooth and liquid.

Morning snack

If you want to keep the snack light and healthy, the individual is advised to take a clementine. That will make up to 35 calories for the day.

Lunch

Since the morning snack was lighter compared to regular days, lunch should be cut back a bit. The consumer can choose to get bread with hummus (keep it low in calories). In addition, about 2 cups of cucumber and white bean salad with basil vinaigrette. This is approximately 352 calories per day.

Cucumber and White Bean Salad

Ingredients

- Basil leaves (1/2 cup)

- Extra virgin olive oil (1/4 cup)

- Vinegar (3 tablespoons)

- Shallot (chopped, one tablespoon)

- Dijon mustard (2 tablespoons)

- Honey (1 tablespoon)

- Salt

- Ground pepper

- Mixed salad greens (10 cups)

- Sodium bean (1 can)

- Grape tomatoes (1 cup)

- Cucumber (1/2)

Directions

1 Add basil, vinegar, shallot, honey, mustard, honey, salt, and pepper in a food processor. Serve the contents with beans, tomato, and cucumber. Toss the salad before serving.

Evening snack

For the evening snack, the individual can eat a plum that contains about 30 calories.

Supper

This meal contains about 490 calories for the day. It consists of about one and a half cups of Mexican cabbage soup and almost 2 cups of black bean salad.

Mexican Cabbage Soup

The soup is real magic for weight loss because it is full of flavor and strengthens the body's defense mechanism. The recipe is suitable for eight people

Ingredients

- Extra virgin olive oil (2 tablespoons)

- Onions (chopped, 2 cups)

- Carrot (chopped, 1 cup)

- Celery (chopped, 1 cup)

- Green pepper (chopped, 1 cup)

- Garlic cloves (4 cloves, chopped)

- Cabbage (sliced, 8 cups)

- Tomato paste (1 tablespoon)

- Adobo sauce (1 tablespoon)

- Cumin (1 tablespoon)

- Coriander (half a teaspoon)

- Chicken stock (4 cups)

- Water (4 cups)

- Low-sodium black beans (2 cans)

- Salt

- Cilantro (half cup)

- Lime juice (2 tablespoons)

- Greek yogurt or avocado as a dressing

Instructions

1. Add oil to a large saucepan and heat it. Then add the contents (celery, onions, carrots, and garlic) and cook for 10-12 minutes.

2. Then add cabbage and cook the mixture. Then add tomato paste, chipotle, cilantro, and the remaining contents and cook for a minute or so. Then add the chicken stock and salt and water. Cover the pan and cook for a while. Finally, garnish the soup with cheese or a garnish of your choice.

Black Bean Salad

Black bean salad is a classic when it comes to taking something light for a picnic.

Ingredients

The following recipe is suitable for four people.

- Sliced onion (half cup)

- Avocado (1)

- Coriander leaves (1/4 cup)

- Lime juice (1/4 cup)

- Olive oil (2 tablespoons)

- Garlic (1 clove)

- Salt

- Salad greens (8 cups)

- Frozen corn (2 cups)

- Grape tomatoes (1 pint)

- Black beans (rinsed)

Instructions

1. Add onions to a bowl of cold water. Add the remaining components to a food processor and blend until smooth. Serve by combining the lettuce creams with the drained mixtures, beans, and onion. Toss to prepare the salad before serving.

Week 2

Day 8

Breakfast

Start the second week with a serving of scrambled eggs with vegetables. It contains about 338 calories for the day.

Morning snack

To keep the snack light and to satisfy the individual, ¼ cup of hummus can be taken along with sliced cucumber. This is approximately 119 calories per day.

Lunch

The individual is advised to make sandwiches with vegetables and hummus. The recipe is mentioned above.

Evening snack

A plum that contains about 30 calories can be taken in the evening as a snack.

Supper

For dinner, the individual can enjoy Greek Kale Salad with Quinoa and Chicken. This meal contains about 302 calories for the day. The recipe for the dish is as follows.

Greek Kale Salad with Quinoa and Chicken

Ingredients

- Kale (finely chopped, 4 cups)

- Grated cooked chicken (1½ cups)

- Quinoa (cooked, 1 cup)

- Red pepper (1/4 cup, roasted)

- Salad dressing with less sodium and sugar

- Feta cheese (to taste)

Directions

Add all the contents in a bowl and mix to make the salad. The individual can add feta cheese to their own taste.

Day 9

Breakfast

The individual can take about 2 cups of Avocado Smoothie. The recipe is mentioned above. It contains about 307 calories for the day.

Morning snack

The individual can take clementine or another similar fruit.

Lunch

For lunch, the individual can have nearly two cups of Mexican cabbage soup, along with a single serving of black bean salad. This is approximately 328 calories per day.

Evening snack

Another light and healthy snack is kiwi and mango with fresh lime zest (about a cup).

Kiwi and Mango with Fresh Lime Zest

Ingredients

- Kiwi (1)

- Mango (1/2 cup)

- Lime zest (1 teaspoon)

Instructions

1 Discard all components and serve the salad at room temperature.

Supper

This meal for the day is relatively heavy, as it has more calories (453). The individual can use a single serving of roasted bean curd with soy lime, colorful roasted vegetables, and citrus vinaigrette as a dressing.

Soy Lime Roasted Tofu

Ingredients

- Drained, water-filled tofu (14 grams)

- Reduced sodium soy sauce (2/3 cup)

- Lime juice (2/3 cup)

- Sesame oil (6 tablespoons)

Instructions

1 Preheat the oven. Add soy sauce, lime juice, and oil in a bowl and then in a bag. Take tofu, cut it into ¼ cubes. Add these cubes to the bag and let them marinate in the refrigerator for about 4 hours, turning the sides of the bag to get the marinade through. Finally, take the tofu out of the bag and add it to a baking sheet and cook until fully cooked to serve.

Colorful roasted vegetables can be a pleasure to the eye as well as the stomach.

Colorful Roasted Vegetables

Ingredients

The recipe can contain about eight servings

- Butternut squash (3 cups)

- Extra virgin olive oil (3 tablespoons)

- Broccoli fleet (4 cups)

- Red pepper (2)

- Red onion (cut into pieces)

- Italian herbs (2 teaspoons)

- Salt

- Pepper

- Balsamic Vinegar (1 tsp)

Instructions

1   Preheat the oven. Add pumpkin and oil to a bowl. Toss around and add them to a baking sheet and roast them. In another bowl, add broccoli, red pepper, onion and Italian herbs, salt, and pepper with the remaining olive oil.

2   Then add vegetables to squash, spread the mixture as a whole on the baking sheet, and sauté for about 20 minutes. Sprinkle vinegar over the vegetables while serving. This dish has a shelf life of almost five days.

Day 10

Breakfast

The individual can take peanut butter with cinnamon for breakfast. It makes up about 290 calories for the day.

Morning snack

A single cup of raspberries can make up for the day's 64 calories.

Lunch

For lunch, the individual can take a serving of chicken and apple cabbage wraps. This is approximately 370 calories. Using kale wraps instead of the bead makes the dish healthier.

Chicken and Apple Cabbage Wraps

Ingredients

- Mayonnaise (1 tablespoon)

- Dijon mustard (1 teaspoon)

- Kale leaves (3)

- Chicken fillet (thinly cooked, 3 grams)

- Red onion (sliced, 6)

- 1 apple (9 slices)

Instructions

1. Place mayonnaise and mustard in a bowl. Add the mixture to the kale leaves. Then cover the leaves with an ounce of chicken, onion, and apple. The required ingredients are for three wraps, so add accordingly.

2. Roll up the sheet into a cover. These can be stored in the refrigerator for a day and then used.

Evening snack

The individual can take any fruit, such as a plum.

Supper

For dinner, the individual may have panko crust mutton chops with Asian slaw. The name of the dish may vary depending on the type of meat used to prepare the dish.

Day 11

Breakfast

Take a single serving of avocado and egg on toast. The bread can be chosen by the individual according to his own taste. It is preferable to be brown bread.

Morning snack

Take 1 cup of raspberries. This is 64 calories per day.

Lunch

This meal contains approximately 302 calories. The individual can enjoy a serving of Greek kale salad with quinoa and chicken.

Evening snack

The individual can enjoy an apple or other fruit.

Supper

For this part of the day, the individual; can enjoy a single serving of salmon and asparagus with lemon-garlic butter sauces and a cup of quinoa.

Salmon and asparagus recipe with lemon garlic butter sauce_is the best combination when it comes to mixing protein and nutrients. It is one of the best healthy dishes that combines fish and vegetables. The recipe is suitable for four people.

Salmon and Asparagus with Lemon Garlic Butter Sauce

Ingredients

- Salmon (1 pound, cut into four portions)

- Asparagus (1 pound)

- Salt

- Pepper

- Butter (3 tablespoons)

- Extra virgin olive oil (1 tablespoon)

- Grated garlic (1/2 teaspoon)

- Lemon zest (1 teaspoon)

- Lemon juice (1 tablespoon)

Instructions

1. Preheat the oven. Place a baking sheet on a pan. Add salmon to the baking sheet on one side and asparagus on the other. Add salt and pepper to both. Add oil, garlic, butter, lemon zest, and juice to a small saucepan and cook until the butter has melted. Then add the mixture to the salmon and asparagus and cook them until the fish is cooked and the asparagus is soft.

Quinoa

Quinoa is a simple side dish that can be prepared with minimal effort. Furthermore, it can be stored for later use.

Ingredients

- Water/Broth (2 cups)

- Quinoa (1 cup)

Instructions

1. Boil the contents and let them simmer until all the water or stock has been observed, and a smooth liquid has formed.

Day 12

Breakfast

The individual can enjoy a single serving of cinnamon toast with peanut butter banana and banana. This works out to about 290 calories for the day.

Morning snack

Snacks can be a mix of dry fruits and vegetables. The individual can take a clementine with 8-9 elements.

Lunch

This meal contains approximately 344 calories. The individual can enjoy a cup of Mexican cabbage soup along with mixed vegetables with citrus vinaigrette.

Evening snack

By keeping proteins under control, the individual can also enjoy a boiled egg with salt and pepper.

Supper

For dinner, the individual can enjoy a single serving of spaghetti and meatballs. This is approximately 408 calories per day.

The recipe for the dish is as follows and serves four.

Spaghetti and Meatballs

Ingredients

- Spaghetti squash (2 pounds)

- Water (2 tablespoons)

- Extra virgin olive oil (2 tablespoons)

- Parsley (half cup)

- Parmesan cheese (half cup)

- Italian herbs (1 teaspoon)

- Onion powder (1 tsp)

- Salt

- Pepper

- Turkey (1 pound)

- Garlic cloves (4, chopped)

- Crushed tomatoes (28 Ounces)

- Rep pepper (crushed, ½ teaspoon)

Instructions

1. Cut the pumpkin in half. Take out the seeds. Microwave the pumpkin for a good 10 minutes until the meat can be easily removed using a fork. Scrape the pumpkin meat into a saucepan and cook it with oil until browned. Stir in half of the parsley.

2. Then remove it and leave it. Combine the remaining parsley, half of the parmesan, Italian herbs, onion powder, salt, and pepper in a bowl. Then add turkey to the bowl to form meatballs. Put one tablespoon of oil in a pan and cook the meatballs until browned. Add garlic and continue cooking. Add the tomato sauce and red pepper to enhance the flavor, along with the remaining Italian spices. Cover the pan and cook the meatballs. Serve the meatballs with the pumpkin and some parmesan.

Day 13

Breakfast

This meal contains approximately 264 calories. The individual can enjoy a low-fat or low-fat Greek yogurt, along with muesli and blueberries.

Morning snack

Take fruits such as clementine or apple.

Lunch

The individual can enjoy a single serving of sandwiches with vegetables and hummus. It contains about 325 calories for the day.

Evening snack

An apple or other food can be taken as an evening snack.

Supper

The individual can enjoy a single serving of zucchini noodles with avocado pest and shrimp. The recipe is listed below.

Zucchini Noodles and Avocado Pesto and Shrimp

Ingredients

- Zucchini (2 pounds)

- Salt

- Avocado (1)

- Basil leaves (1 cup)

- Unsalted pistachios (1/4 cup)

- Lemon juice (2 tablespoons)

- Ground pepper

- Extra virgin olive oil (2 tablespoons)

- Garlic (3 cloves)

- Shrimp (1 pound)

- Spices (1-2 tablespoon)

Instructions

1. Make zucchini noodles by cutting them into long strips lengthwise. Place the noodles in the bar and drain in water. As the noodles drain, create a past consisting of avocado, lemon juice, basil, and the rest of the contents. Add oil to obtain a smooth mixture. In a large skillet, add oil and cook the shrimp. Season the shrimp. Once seasoned, move them to a large bowl. After individual preparation, both items combine and serve.

Day 14

Breakfast

Take a single serving of avocado and egg on toast. The bread can be an individual's choice depending on whether the individual likes white or brown bread and is gluten intolerant or not.

Morning snack

Any fruit can be taken as a morning snack.

Lunch

Take about 2 cups for tomato, cucumber, and white bean salad with basil vinaigrette along with basil, bread, and hummus. This is approximately 378 calories per day.

Evening snack

Plum can be taken in the evening.

Supper

The individual can enjoy a single serving of fish with coconut with shallot sauce, quinoa, and some citrus vinaigrette. This will make up to 458 calories per day.

The recipe is suitable for four people.

Fish with Coconut and Shallot Sauce, Quinoa, and Some Citrus Vinaigrette

Ingredients

- Garlic cloves (3, chopped)

- Salt

- Extra virgin olive oil (2 tablespoons)

- Dried thyme (2 teaspoons)

- Ground pepper

- Fish cut in four portions (red snapper)

- Chopped shallot (2 Tbsp.)

- Coconut milk (1 cup)

- Lime wedges

Instructions

1   Preheat the oven. Mash/mix the garlic with salt into a paste. Then combine it with oil, thyme, and pepper. Now put the fish in a pan and spread the made marinade on top. Cook the fish for 6-9 minutes. To make the sauce, take oil and add shallot. Add coconut milk and let the mixture simmer to make a paste. Add the pasta to the fish and serve with the lime wedges.

It is recommended to prepare and store dressings such as lemon tahini and citrus vinaigrette. This makes dieting even easier.

It can be noted that the individual should consume about 1200-1500 calories per day. The individual observes a diet full of vegetables, rich in antioxidants and nutrients—a lot of fiber and few calories and carbohydrates. Furthermore, the berries consumed regularly help the consumer to maintain the inflammation. Inflammation is one of the main reasons for obesity (weight gain). Of the many diseases that can act as a side effect of inflammation, obesity is one of them. Following a strict and healthy diet not only helps the individual control the disease but also helps the individual lose weight. By following the diet, the individual can lose about 4 pounds in 2 weeks.

Losing weight is not only good for a person, but also for the individual because the individual is more confident and leads a better life.

Cookbook—Some Ideas for Recipes

Ideas for Meals

- **Food for breakfast:** Chia bowl. Breakfast smoothie, oatmeal.

- **Food for lunch:** soup, grilled salmon, salad with quinoa, and vegetables.

- **Food for snacks:** apples, nut butter, fresh blueberry salad, walnuts, guacamole, chia seed pudding.

Some Recipes for an Anti-Inflammatory Diet

The following are some recipes from an anti-inflammatory diet that are not only simple and delicious, but also help strengthen the immune system, reduce inflammation, and reduce weight.

Cherry Coconut Porridge

Ingredients

- Cups of oats

- Four tablespoons of Chia Seeds

- 4 cups of coconut milk

- Tablespoons of raw cocoa

- A pinch of Stevia

- Coconut curls

- Cherries

- Dark chocolate chips

- Maple syrup

Instructions

1. First, combine the oats, coconut milk, cocoa, chia, and stevia in a pan. Now the ingredients bring to a boil over medium heat.

2. After these are cooked, simmer over low heat until the oats are cooked through. Then put these ingredients in a bowl and cover with coconut shavings, cherries, dark chocolate shavings, and maple syrup to your liking and taste.

Thai Pumpkin Soup

Ingredients

- Two tablespoons of red curry paste

- Cups of chicken or vegetable stock

- Two cans of pumpkin puree (15 grams each)

- One and ¾ cup of coconut milk

- 1 large red chili pepper

- Coriander for garnish

Instructions

1 Cook the curry paste in a large saucepan over medium heat for about a minute or until the paste becomes fragrant. Now add the stock and pumpkin puree and stir.

2 Cook the soup for about 3 minutes or until it starts to boil. Then add the coconut milk and cook the soup until hot. Now pour the soup into bowls and garnish with the reserved coconut milk and sliced red chilies. Garnish with coriander leaves if you like it.

Curry Potatoes With Poached Eggs

Ingredients

- Russet potatoes

- 1 inch of fresh ginger

- Cloves of garlic

- 1 tablespoon of olive oil

- Two tablespoons of curry powder

- Canned tomato sauce

- Four large eggs

- ½ bunch of fresh cilantro

Instructions

1 Wash the potatoes thoroughly and cut them into cubes. Place the diced potatoes in a large saucepan and cover with water.

2 Now cover the pot with a lid and bring it to a boil over high heat until cooked. Now drain the boiled potatoes in a sieve. Start cooking the sauce while the potatoes are cooking. Peel the ginger. Grate about an inch of ginger using a grater. Then chop the garlic. Now add the ginger, garlic, and olive oil to a large and deep skillet.

3 Fry the ginger and garlic for about 1 to 2 minutes over medium heat or until getting soften and fragrant. Now also add the curry powder to the pan and cook for

another minute to roast the herbs. After sautéing, add the tomato sauce and stir well to combine. Put the heat on medium heat and heat the sauce. Add salt if necessary and add more if you want. Add the boiled and drained potatoes to the pan and stir well to add the sauce. Add some tablespoons of water if the mixture appears dry or pasty.

4   Now make four small pits in the potato mixture and crack one egg in each dip. Then cover the skillet with a lid and let the curry potatoes come to a boil. Simmer the eggs in the sauce for about 6-10 minutes, or until tender. Place them in the latter with chopped fresh cilantro.

Raspberry Smoothie

Ingredients

- 1 pitted avocado and peeled

- 3/4 cup of orange juice

- 3/4 cup of raspberry juice

- 1/2 cup of raspberries

Instructions

1 Add all listed ingredients in a blender and mix well.

Mediterranean Tuna Salad

Ingredients

- Two cans of 5 oz. tuna packed in water and keep drained

- 1/4 cup of mayonnaise

- 1/4 cup chopped kalamata or mixed olives

- Tablespoons of chopped red onion

- Two tablespoons chopped fire-roasted red pepper

- Two tablespoons chopped fresh basil

- 1 tablespoon of capers

- One tablespoon of fresh lemon juice

- Salt and pepper to taste

- Large vine tomatoes

Directions

1 Place all ingredients except tomatoes in a large bowl and stir well to combine. Cut the tomatoes into sixths without cutting all the way through and then carefully pry them open. Spoon the Mediterranean tuna salad mixture into the center of the tomatoes and serve.

Slow Cooker Turkey Chili

Ingredients

- 1 tablespoon of olive oil

- 1 pound 99% lean turkey

- 1 medium onion chopped

- 1 red pepper, chopped

- One yellow bell pepper chopped

- Two cans of 15 oz. tomato sauce

- Two cans of 15 oz. petite chopped tomatoes

- Two cans of 15 oz. black beans, rinsed and drained

- Two cans of 15 oz. red beans, rinsed and drained

- One jar 16 oz. deli sliced jalapeno peppers tamed and let them drain.

- 1 cup of frozen corn

- Tablespoons of chili powder

- 1 tablespoon of cumin

- Salt and black pepper to taste

- Optional toppings of green onions, grated cheese, avocado, sour cream or Greek yogurt

Instructions

1 First, heat the oil in a skillet over medium heat. Now put

the turkey in the pan and cook until brown. Now pour the turkey into a slow cooker. Then add the onion, bell pepper, tomato sauce, diced tomatoes, beans, jalapeños, corn, chili powder, and cumin to the stove as well.

2   Stir and season with salt and pepper. Then cover and cook on high heat for 4 hours or on low heat for 6 hours. Serve it with toppings if you like.

Gingerbread Oatmeal

Ingredients

- Cups of water

- 1 cup of steel-cut oats

- 1 and ½ tbsp. ground cinnamon

- 1/4 teaspoon. ground coriander

- 1/4 teaspoon. ground cloves

- 1/4 teaspoon. ground ginger

- 1/4 teaspoon. of ground allspice

- 1/8 tsp. ground nutmeg

- 1/4 teaspoon. ground cardamom

- Maple syrup to taste

Instructions

1 Take the oats and cook them according to the packer's directions. Also, add the spices when adding the oats to the water. When the oats have finished cooking, add maple syrup to taste.

Kale Caesar Salad with Grilled Chicken Wrap

Ingredients

- Thinly sliced grilled chicken

- Cups of kale cut into bite-sized pieces

- 1 cup quartered cherry tomatoes

- ¾ cup of finely grated Parmesan cheese

- ½ cloudy egg that is cooked for about 1 minute

- 1 clove of minced garlic

- 1/2 teaspoon of Dijon mustard

- 1 teaspoon of honey or agave

- 1/8 cup of fresh lemon juice

- 1/8 cup of olive oil

- Freshly ground black pepper and Kosher salt to taste

- Lavash flatbreads or two large tortillas

Instructions

1 Mix half of a confused egg, minced garlic, mustard, honey, lemon juice, and olive oil in a bowl. Beat them until you've formed a dressing consistency. Season to taste with salt and pepper. Now add the kale, chicken and cherry tomatoes and toss through the dressing and ¼ cup of grated parmesan.

2 Now spread the two lavash flatbreads and spread the

salad evenly over the two pieces of bread and sprinkle with ¼ cup of parmesan cheese. Roll up the wraps and cut in half.

Baked Tilapia with Pecan Rosemary Topping

Ingredients

- 1/3 cup chopped raw pecans

- 1/3 cup whole-wheat panko breadcrumbs

- Two teaspoons chopped fresh rosemary

- Half a teaspoon of coconut palm sugar / brown sugar

- 1/8 teaspoon of salt

- One pinch of cayenne pepper

- 1 and 1/2 teaspoon of olive oil

- 1 egg white

- Four each 4-ounce tilapia fillets

Instructions

1   Preheat your oven to 350 degrees F. Take a small baking dish and add pecans, breadcrumbs, rosemary, coconut palm sugar, salt, and cayenne pepper to stir them together. Now add the olive oil and mix to cover the prepared pecan mixture. Bake the mixture until the pecan mixture is lightly golden brown for about 7 to 8 minutes.

2   Now increase the heat to 400 degrees F. Now coat a large glass baking dish with cooking spray. Then beat the egg white in a shallow dish. Work one tilapia at a

time, covering each side lightly by dipping the fish in the egg white mixture and then in the pecan mixture. Then place the fillets in the prepared baking dish. Add the remaining pecan mixture on top of the tilapia fillets. Now bake until the tilapia is cooked for about 10 minutes and serve.

Rhubarb, Apple and Ginger Muffins

Ingredients

- 1/2 cup almond flour (ground almonds)
- 1/4 cup of unrefined raw sugar
- Two tablespoons finely chopped crystallized ginger
- One tablespoon of ground flaxseed flour
- 1/2 cup of buckwheat flour
- 1/4 cup of fine brown rice flour
- Two tablespoons of organic corn flour
- Teaspoons of gluten-free baking powder
- 1/2 teaspoon of ground cinnamon
- 1/2 teaspoon of ground ginger
- A good pinch of fine sea salt
- 1 cup of chopped rhubarb
- One small apple, peeled, cored and cut into small cubes
- 1/3 cup + 1 tablespoon of rice or almond milk
- 1/4 cup of olive oil
- 1 large free-range egg
- 1 teaspoon of vanilla extract

Instructions

1   First, preheat your oven to 180C / 350C. Grease the

eight 1/3 cups of 180 ml muffin tins with paper tins. Now put the almond meal, sugar, ginger, and flaxseed flour in a medium bowl. Then sift the flour, baking powder, and spices and beat to combine evenly.

2   Now stir in the rhubarb and apple to cover the flour mixture. Take another smaller bowl and whisk together the milk, oil, egg, and vanilla before pouring into the dry mixture and stirring until just combined.

3   Now spread the batter evenly over the tins or cartons and bake for about 20-25 minutes or until they have risen, golden on the edges, and when a skewer is inserted in the center, it comes out clean.

4   Then take them out of the oven and set them aside for about 5 minutes before transferring them to an open tray or wiring rack to cool further. Eat them warm or at room temperature. These are best eaten on the day of baking; however, they can be stored in an airtight container for about 2-3 days.

Winter Fruit Salad with Agave-Pomegranate Vinaigrette

Ingredients

- Cut 4 Fuyu persimmons into 1-inch cubes

- Bosch pears and cut into 1-inch cubes

- 1 cup of grapes and cut into halves or quarters when large

- 3/4 cup pecans and cut them in half lengthwise to make strips

Dressing

- 1 T extra virgin olive oil

- 1 T peanut oil

- 1 Pomegranate-flavored vinegar

- T agave nectar or sweetener of your choice

- A pinch of salt to taste

Directions

1 First, whisk together the dressing ingredients so that the flavors can blend well while you cut the fruit. Now cut the grapes, persimmon, and pears into pieces of the same size and place them in a plastic bowl. Then toss the fruits with dressing. Toss them with pieces of pecan just before serving.

Italian Style Stuffed Red Peppers

Ingredients

- 1 pound of lean ground turkey

- Red peppers

- Cups of spaghetti sauce

- One teaspoon of basil or oregano herbs

- 1 teaspoon of garlic powder

- 1/2 teaspoon of salt and pepper

- 1/2 cup frozen chopped spinach

- Grated Parmesan cheese + 6 tbsp. extra for garnish over each pepper

- Optional one teaspoon of low-calorie sweetener of your choice to put in the sauce

Instructions

1   First, preheat your oven to 450 degrees. Then line the baking sheet with foil and cover with non-stick cooking spray. Now wash the red peppers and cut around the stem to remove it. Then remove the stems. Take the bell pepper and cut it in half lengthwise and then remove the seeds and ribs from the bell peppers. Place the peppers on the baking tin. Cook the ground turkey in a large nonstick pan over medium heat. Stir and grate the turkey while cooking. When the turkey is cooked, then add the

sauce and herbs in the pan. Stir and keep cooking until the turkey is cooked through. Now add the spinach and parmesan and stir them well until everything is well combined. Spoon 1/2 cup of the turkey mixture into each pepper.

2 Then sprinkle one tablespoon of Parmesan cheese over each pepper. Bake them for about 20-30 minutes or until the cheese is melted and lightly golden brown. Remove from the oven and enjoy.

Buckwheat and Ginger Granola

Ingredients

- 1 cup of buckwheat

- Rolled oats that are gluten-free

- 1 cup of shelled sunflower seeds

- 1 cup of pumpkin seeds

- 1 and 1/2 cup pitted dates

- 1 cup of apple sauce that is unsweetened

- Coconut oil

- Raw cocoa powder

- One piece of 1-inch ginger root

Instructions

1 First, preheat your oven to 180C. Now put the oats, buckwheat, and seeds in a large mixing bowl and stir well. Now add the coconut oil, dates, and apple sauce to a pan and let them simmer until the dates are nice and soft. While the dates are cooked, peel the ginger and grate on a plate. After it has been grated, mix it in the date pan.

2 When the dates are soft, put them together with the other ingredients, including grated ginger, melted coconut oil, and apple sauce, in a blender with the raw cocoa powder

and mix well until smooth. Then pour this mixture over the buckwheat, oat, and seed mix and stir well so that everything is covered. Now grease a large baking tray with coconut oil before spreading the granola over it— Bake for about 45 minutes.

3   After the first fifteen minutes, remove the trays from the oven and stir everything well so that the top does not burn, and put it in the oven every five to ten minutes the rest of the time. When it is nice and crispy, remove the granola from the oven. Let the granola cool before storing it in an airtight container.

Roasted Red Pepper and Sweet Potato Soup

Ingredients

- Tablespoons of olive oil

- Medium onions

- One jar of roasted red pepper, chopped and liquid

- One can of diced green chilies

- Teaspoons of cumin powder

- 1 teaspoon of salt

- 1 teaspoon of ground coriander

- 4 cups of peeled and diced sweet potatoes

- Cups of vegetable stock

- Two tablespoons chopped fresh cilantro

- One tablespoon of lemon juice

- Diced cream cheese

Instructions

1. Take a large stockpot or a Dutch oven and heat the olive oil over medium heat. Add the onion and cook until soft. Now add in the red chilies, green chilies, cumin, salt, and coriander, then cook them for about 1-2 minutes. Then stir in the reserved juice of the roasted red pepper, sweet potatoes, and vegetable stock.

2. Bring it to a boil and reduce the heat, and cover. Cook it

until the potatoes are tender for about 10 to 15 minutes. Stir in the coriander and lemon juice and let the soup cool slightly. Then put half of the soup together with the cream cheese in a blender and mix until smooth. Add the mixed mixture back to the stockpot and heat through. Season with extra salt if necessary.

Lemon Herb Salmon and Zucchini

Ingredients

- Four chopped zucchini

- Tablespoons of olive oil

- Freshly ground black pepper and Kosher salt to taste

- Two tablespoons of packed brown sugar

- Two tablespoons of freshly squeezed lemon juice

- One tablespoon of Dijon mustard

- Cloves of minced garlic

- 1/2 teaspoon of dried dill

- 1/2 teaspoon of dried oregano

- 1/4 teaspoon of dried thyme

- 1/4 teaspoon of dried rosemary

- Four salmon fillets of 5 grams each

- Two tablespoons chopped fresh parsley leaves

Directions

1 First, preheat your oven to 400 degrees F. Then take a baking tray and lightly coat it or cover it with nonstick cooking spray. Take a small bowl and whisk together brown sugar, lemon juice, Dijon, garlic, dill, oregano, thyme, and rosemary. Season the ingredients to taste with salt and pepper. Set it aside. In a single layer, place

the zucchini on the prepared baking sheet. Now sprinkle it with olive oil and season with salt and pepper. Then add the salmon in a single layer and brush each salmon fillet with the spice mixture.

2   Place them in the oven and cook until the fish flakes easily with a fork for about 16-18 minutes. Serve immediately after garnishing with parsley.

Baby Spinach and Frittata Mushroom

Ingredients

- Six eggs

- 1/4 cup of milk

- 1 cup of grated cheddar cheese

- 1 thinly sliced onion

- Sliced white mushrooms

- Tablespoons of butter

- Cups of young spinach

- Salt and pepper to taste

Instructions

1   Place the rack in the middle and preheat the oven to 180 ° C. Now, butter a square baking dish of 20 cm and set it aside. Take a large bowl and combine eggs and milk with a whisk, then add the cheese. Season the beaten eggs and milk to taste with salt and pepper. Set the bowl aside.

2   Take a large non-stick skillet, heat the butter and fry the onions and mushrooms over medium heat. Season the onions with salt and pepper. Now add spinach and continue to cook for about 1 minute, stirring constantly. Then pour the mushroom mixture into the egg mixture.

3   Stir well and pour into a baking dish. Bake for about 25 minutes or until light brown and puffy. Cut your frittata into four squares and remove them from the bowl. Place it on a plate, and it is ready to be served hot or cold.

Smoked Salmon Potato Tartine

Ingredients

- One large peeled and grated red-brown potato

- Tablespoons of clarified butter

- Kosher salt

- Freshly ground black pepper

- Soft goat cheese

- 1 and 1/2 tablespoon finely chopped chives

- 1/2 finely chopped garlic clove

- Zest of half a lemon

- Thinly sliced smoked salmon

- Two tablespoons of drained capers

- Tablespoons of chopped red onion

- 1/2 finely chopped hard-boiled egg

- Finely chopped chives

Instructions

2   Take a small bowl and combine the goat cheese, lemon zest, and garlic. Season these ingredients to taste with salt and pepper. Then gently stir in the fresh chives and set aside. Now season the chopped red onion and the hard-boiled egg with salt.

3   Work quickly because the potato will oxidize quickly. Grate the potato into a large one with the large holes of a grater. Then squeeze the potatoes over the sink to remove any excess liquid. Season with salt and pepper and scoop. Heat the clarified butter in a 20 to 30 cm non-stick frying pan over medium heat. When it is hot, add the grated potato and shape them into a large circle with a spatula.

4   Cover and cook gently for about 8-10 minutes or until the bottom is golden brown. Then carefully turn to the other side and cook for another 8-10 minutes or until golden brown and crispy. Transfer it to a cooling rack and let it cool until it is barely lukewarm or at room temperature.

5   Once the potato pie has cooled, spread the goat cheese mixture over it. Place the smoked salmon directly on top and sprinkle with the red onions, the hard-boiled egg, and the capers. Garnish with freshly cut chives and cut into wedges. Serve immediately.

Sweet Potato Black Bean Burgers

Ingredients

- 1/2 cup of quinoa

- One can of black beans and keep rinsed and drained

- 1 large sweet potato

- 1/2 cup diced red onion

- Cloves of minced garlic

- 1/2 cup chopped cilantro

- 1/2 seeds and diced jalapeno

- 1 teaspoon of cumin

- Two teaspoons of spicy Cajun spices

- 1/4 cup gluten-free oat flour

- Salt and pepper to taste

- Olive or coconut oil

- Six whole wheat hamburger buns

- Brussels sprouts

For Avocado Cilantro Cream

- 1/2 large diced ripe avocado

- 1/4 cup low-fat sour cream or regular Greek yogurt

- Tablespoons chopped cilantro

- 1 teaspoon of lime juice

- Splash of hot sauce

- Salt to taste

Instructions

1   First, rinse the quinoa with cold water in a gauze strainer. Take a medium saucepan and bring 1 cup of water to a boil. Now add the quinoa and bring the mixture to a boil. Cover the pan, reduce the heat to low, and simmer for about 15 minutes. Now remove from the heat and mix quinoa with a fork. Then place the quinoa in a large bowl and set aside to cool for about 10 minutes. Now prick the sweet potato several times with a fork and place it in the microwave until soft and cooked. Be careful not to overcook the sweet potato, or it will harden.

2   Now remove the skin when you have finished cooking and after it has cooled down. In a food processor bowl, add the beans, boiled sweet potato, red onion, cilantro, garlic, cumin, Cajun seasoning, pulse, and mix until almost smooth, occasionally scraping down the sides of the processor if necessary.

3   Then put the mixture in a bowl and combine it with cooked quinoa. Add salt and pepper to taste.

4   Now mix enough oat bran/oat flour so that you can form patties. Divide into six patties and place on baking paper on a baking tray. Let them cool for at least 30 minutes to allow patties to bind together.

5   Place sour cream, diced avocado, cilantro, and lime juice in a food processor bowl. Process them until smooth. Add salt to taste and refrigerate until ready to serve burgers.

6   Heat the skillet over medium heat and spray the pan with cooking spray. Place the patties in the pan and bake for about 3-4 minutes on each side or until golden brown. Serve them with sandwiches, Brussels sprouts, crema, and the desired toppings.

Gluten-Free Pancakes

Ingredients

- 1 and 3/4 cups xanthan gum-free gluten-free flour mix

- 1/4 teaspoon of Kosher salt

- Three beaten eggs at room temperature

- Tablespoons of melted and cooled unsalted butter

- Cups of milk, should be at room temperature

Instructions

1   Take a large bowl and add the flour mix and salt, and beat well. Take a separate, small bowl and put the eggs, butter, and milk together and beat them. Now make a small well in the center of the flour and add the wet ingredients. Then beat again until thoroughly combined. You will see the batter thicken a little while you knock.

2   The batter should have a consistency of half and half. Then put the batter in a large measuring cup with a spout. Heat a heavy-bottomed, nonstick skillet over medium heat for about 2 minutes. Cook the pancakes on one side of the pan and turn them over and cook the other side as well.

3   Repeat this process with the remaining batter and continue to stack the finished pancakes on top. The pancakes should be well covered with a damp towel, and

they should be kept at room temperature for about 2 hours or until you want to serve them. Or you can wrap them tightly in a freezer-safe container and let them freeze until ready to use.

Red Lentils and Pumpkin Curry Stew

Ingredients

- One teaspoon of extra virgin olive oil

- 1 sweet chopped onion

- Three cloves of minced garlic,

- One tablespoon of superior quality curry powder

- 1 cardboard stock

- 1 cup of red lentils

- Cups of cooked pumpkin

- 1 cup of greens of your choice

- Freshly grated ginger to taste

- Kosher salt & black pepper to taste

Instructions

1. Take a large pan and add extra virgin oil, chopped onion, and chopped garlic. Sauté them over medium heat for about 5 minutes. Now add the curry powder to the pan and cook for a few more minutes. Now add the stock and lentils and bring them to a boil.

2. Then reduce the heat and almost cook for about 10 minutes. Add the cooked pumpkin and vegetables of your choice. Cook them for about 5-8 minutes on medium heat and season with salt and pepper and add some freshly grated ginger to taste.

Stuffed Peppers With Turkey and Quinoa

Ingredients

- Large yellow peppers

- Extra lean ground turkey

- 1 cup diced mushrooms

- 1/4 cup diced sweet onion

- 1 cup chopped fresh spinach

- Two teaspoons minced garlic

- 1 cup tomato sauce

- 1 cup chicken stock

- 1 cup dry quinoa

- Cheese of your choice

Instructions

1   Take a small saucepan and start the quinoa and cook according to the directions in the package. While the quinoa is cooking, fry the vegetables in a pan with some butter or olive oil. Then, after about 5 minutes, add the ground turkey and garlic to the vegetables. Cook them over medium heat. If the turkey is almost cooked, add then the tomato sauce and about half of the chicken stock. Simmer until the turkey is fully cooked, and some of the excess liquid is done. Preheat the oven to 400.

2   While the turkey mixture is simmering, prepare your peppers.

Cut the peppers in half and also remove the stem and seeds. Spray a baking tin with cooking spray and place the cut peppers in the pan with the open side up. Once the quinoa is done cooking, then add it to the pan with the turkey and vegetables. Stir them well and then fill all the peppers with the mixture. If you plan to use the cheese, cover the peppers with just enough cheese to barely cover the mixture. Then pour the leftover chicken stock into the bottom of the pan and around the peppers and not over it. Cover them with foil and bake at 400 for about 30-35 minutes. These are ready to serve and eat hot.

Frequently Asked Questions about the Anti-Inflammatory Diet

Should Everything Be Prepared From Scratch in an Anti-Inflammatory Diet?

No, it is not always important to select and create everything from scratch. In fact, it would be great if you plan to buy packaged food and prepare a meal. While there is only one thing you should care about is to always analyze the ingredients before purchasing. Food with a minimally processed ratio would be best.

Should All Dairy Products Be Removed From the Diet?

Not every dairy product causes inflammation. And unlike inflammation, many dairy products have an anti-inflammatory effect on certain people. For example, yogurt supports intestinal health and reduces inflammation. Although saturated fats cause inflammation, they should be taken in moderation. If someone has an allergic effect on dairy products, he/she should not use them because they cause inflammation as an allergic reaction.

Should Nightshade Vegetables Be Avoided?

The nightshade vegetables like potatoes, eggplants, pepper, and tomatoes are said to cause arthritis inflammation. It has not been proven by the research, so do not remove these vegetables.

Because these vegetables are filled with anti-inflammatory elements. However, if you have an allergic inflammation for a particular vegetable, avoid using only that specific vegetable.

Is a Glass of Wine Acceptable?

During the detox and recovery phase, any nutritional element or any food can cause inflammation in the body, so it is best not to consume any alcoholic drinks during this period.

However, after this period, you can add a drink to your meal. If you drink wine, beer, or a drink in a moderate way, these can even be part of your anti-inflammatory diet.

Are the Artificial Sweeteners a Healthy and a Good Substitute for the Sugar?

The artificial sweeteners are mainly produced in laboratories. These synthetic elements can cause an allergic reaction in some people and cause inflammation. These are also not tested, and no good research is done on them, so it is always a doubt whether they are safe or not. However, if you still want to use artificial sweeteners, you can use the ones that are low in calories and vegetables. Because using a sweetener made from plants is always a safe and healthy option than a chemical lab-made sweetener.

Conclusion

An anti-inflammatory diet is best to reduce chronic inflammation, physical and mental health, and to lose weight. This is the story of a person who has tried the anti-inflammatory diet and how it has helped reduce inflammation.

The person develops sciatica after his/her sacrum is turned out of alignment. While the alignment returned to normal, problems like nerve pain with pain and numbness got worse by the day. Everything was tried, from the osteopathy to the pain reliever, but nothing worked. Then after some research, the person tried the anti-inflammatory diet. In just a month, it showed results, and the pain was reduced.

Because chronic inflammation plays a key role in overcoming various diseases, and it is extremely harmful to the health of the person, an anti-inflammatory diet helps to increase all of these risks and concerns. By properly starting and maintaining an anti-inflammatory diet, many heart conditions and health risks are reduced, the body recovers and begins to function properly, and it is also very helpful in reducing body weight, apart from physical health. All the waste material from the body is excreted from time to time, and the proper blood flow from the heart to all parts of the body is regulated. An anti-inflammatory diet is easy to follow and maintain. It is best for everyone, be it heart or diabetes patients.